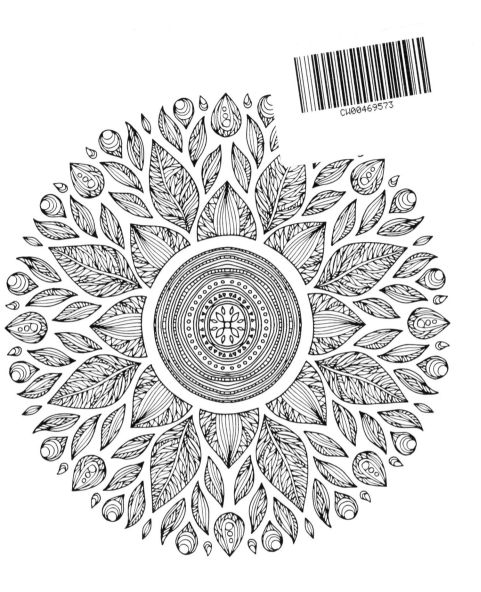

YOGA FOR WITCHES

Sarah Robinson

Medical disclaimer

The information provided in this book and other materials online are for reference and not a substitute for medical advice or direct guidance of a qualified yoga instructor. Please practice with care and compassion for yourself. The author and publishers assume no responsibility or liability for any injuries or losses that may result from practicing yoga or witchcraft.

Not all yoga poses are suitable for everyone. Practicing under the direct supervision and guidance of a qualified instructor can help determine what poses are suitable for you. Always, if in any doubt, consult with your healthcare provider before practicing yoga or any other exercise program.

Published by Womancraft Publishing, 2020
www.womancraftpublishing.com

ISBN 978-1-910559-55-0
Yoga for Witches is also available in ebook format: ISBN 978-1-910559-54-3

Cover design and typesetting by Lucent Word, www.lucentword.com
Cover image © Adriana Hristova
Yoga sequence images © Lisa R. Nelson (PainterLisa.com)
Chakra images: Trikona/Shutterstock.com
Mandala image: Benjavisa Ruangvaree Art/Shutterstock.com

Womancraft Publishing is committed to sharing powerful new women's voices, through a collaborative publishing process. We are proud to midwife this work, however the story, the experiences and the words are the author's alone. A percentage of Womancraft Publishing profits are invested back into the environment reforesting the tropics (via TreeSisters) and forward into the community: providing books for girls in developing countries, and affordable libraries for red tents and women's groups around the world.

Praise for
Yoga for Witches

Yoga for Witches is a treat for yoginis and witches alike.
The book is a practical friend for everyone who's looking to integrate our indigenous wisdom of witchery and earth-based connection with the spiritual practices of yoga. Sarah Robinson offers a valuable, simple guide for the curious yogi or the beginning witch. This is a great introduction to the fundamental links between an embodied cyclical practice of everyday witchcraft and the most straightforward of yoga techniques.

Uma Dinsmore-Tuli PhD, author of *Yoni Shakti: a woman's guide to power and freedom through yoga and tantra*, co-founder of The Yoga Nidra Network and Santosa Eco Yoga Camps

Yoga for Witches is smart, well written and its subject is a welcome change and unique contribution to the ever expanding literature of contemporary Witchcraft. Most importantly, the author's genuine and warm-hearted spirit welcomes and encourages the reader to discover, explore and cultivate a life filled with real magic.

Phyllis Curott, Wiccan Priestess, activist attorney, internationally best-selling author of *Book of Shadows, Wicca Made Easy, The Witches Wisdom Tarot,* and Vice Chair Emerita, Parliament of the World's Religions

Yoga for Witches combines two ancient traditions in a fascinating and readable way. An essential book for the modern seeker looking to bring their faith and spiritual yoga practice together in new and inspiring ways.

Alice B. Grist, author of *Dirty and Divine*

Yoga for Witches is a beautifully written book that blends yoga with the art of witchcraft, tapping into natural magic that happens both on and off the yoga mat. Sarah gently shows you how you can enhance your life through Eastern wisdom and Western magical practice, throwing in goddesses, rituals and practical suggestions along the way. It's a perfect book for yogis who are curious about witchcraft as well as witches looking for a deeper connection to their craft.

Lyn Thurman, author of *Goddess Rising* and *The Inner Goddess Revolution*

If I ever take up yoga, this is the book I'm going to use.

Paula Brackston, author of *The Witch's Daughter*

In Yoga for Witches Sarah Robinson has found a delightful balance as she simultaneously demystifies and honors the mystery inherent in both yoga and witchcraft. This book is rich with information about both traditions, yet it never overwhelms the reader. Deeply scholarly and yet totally accessible, Yoga for Witches awakens the magic within each one of us.

Gina Martin, author of *Sisters of the Solstice Moon*

A 'must-read' for all the closet yoga-witches out there needing the tools and motivations to proudly reclaim our herstory as healers, wise women, goddesses, yogis, priestesses and oracles.

Tamara Pitelen, founder of Blue Dea Books, author, energy healer and yoga instructor

I have longed for a book like this to be written! I've noticed many correlations between witchcraft and yoga and Sarah puts them in words that are eloquent and knowledgeable. The blend between the craft of a Witch and the deep-rooted history of Yoga brings, through the many well-crafted spiritual practices in this book, the reader to stay grounded through the breath, movement and to be mindful of the many cycles we, as witches follow.

Katie Smith, astrologer and designer of the Urban Witchery® Planner

For Mum, The Finest Kitchen Witch

CONTENTS

Am I then supposed to be saying that Yoga is merely the handmaiden of Magick, or that Magick has no higher function than to supplement Yoga? By no means. It is the cooperation of lovers... The practices of Yoga are almost essential to success in Magick.
Aleister Crowley

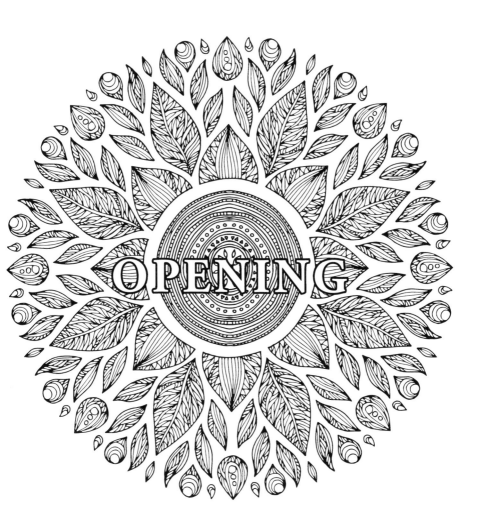

"*Yoga for witches?*" my yoga student looked at me with genuine concern. "Are you sure you want to use the word *witch?*"

By her own admission, she loved magic, or *muti* as she called it in her native tongue. But she struggled with the word witch…there were too many negative connotations. She seemed so concerned about me using the word in my title, that it would put people off, that people would be offended or angry.

"But don't you see," I replied, "that's exactly why I have to use that word, it's our word, and it's been taken from us. It's been twisted and made this negative thing. I'm reclaiming it, and it's okay if that makes us feel a little uncomfortable. I'm prepared to do my tiny part of reclaiming this."

"So, if you're a witch…would you ever work with healing?" she continued.

"I already do," I replied.

Yoga is my healing tool of choice. You might work through your own healing with herbs, meditation, dance, crafting, connection with nature, tarot, crystals… Every witch will use her particular skills and knowledge to heal herself, her loved ones, and if we are lucky, she will share her gifts with others too.

Find Your Magic on the Mat

"Find your magic on the mat" is a phrase I have often used in the yoga classes I teach. It's a phrase that brings together my two favourite spiritual practices: yoga and witchcraft. These are not practices that many people would associate, and so this book was born from my desire to connect and highlight the many beautiful similarities between magical practice and yoga.

Yoga is an embodied spiritual practice: moving the body, using intention and focused breathing to guide our movements. Yoga is a kind of ritual, each yoga asana (pose) not only moves the physical body but also the body's energy in its various forms. Witchcraft is, well, not so very different: a spiritual practice, that involves intention and focus. But also, a practice of creation and connection to spiritual and natural realms and cycles.

Magical pioneers throughout history have used meditation (and yoga) to focus and delve deeper into the process of creating magic. The goal of *Yoga for Witches* is to let this path be a two-way street.

Some of us already have an idea of what a witch is…and what yoga is…and it may be that we cannot yet see how the two would ever belong together. During the next few pages, we will explore the original meanings and intentions of both terms, and see what a natural fit they are.

Uniting yoga with witchcraft allows us to create tangible experiences with the energy that connects our universe. *Yoga for Witches* is an exploration of how these two spiritual disciplines can be combined and explored to find greater peace, power and magic in our lives. This book will guide you through the basic principles and some more advanced techniques found in both witchcraft and yoga, illuminating connections that we may not have previously considered.

My Journey

Yoga is something I have done since the age of seven. I've practised many styles in many cities around the world. While I didn't have a witchy upbringing, I was a member of the Woodcraft Folk (a pagan version of guides and scouts) and…*whisper* I was a Morris dancer! So a connection with the natural world, folk traditions and a sprinkling of paganism have shimmered through my childhood. Not long after my first yoga class, I purchased a CD for meditation – it was called *Ocean Dreams*. And I started a regular meditation practice that continues to this day. I also kept a modest box of (what I considered, to be) magical items. A small box of crystals and stones I picked up at a summer fair, an old ornate button with blue stones in it and a book of spells entitled *How to Turn Your Ex-boyfriend into a Toad*. But mainly the spells and rituals I played with, I made up myself. This continues to be true, I've never been great at strictly following recipes or rules.

I have taken on more conscious learning over the last few years. I am studying to become a Priestess at the Glastonbury Goddess Temple (specifically honouring the Celtic Goddess Brigid). And am delving deeper into many practices: pagan, druid and witchcraft. I now have my own *Book of Shadows* (see Chapter 6) and have taken every opportunity to learn from other witches. It's been a meandering path to being what you might call a Yoga Witch.

I am growing to really love this as a term, as it encapsulates to me the ancient etymological roots from which the word *witch* originated – namely *wicca* and *wicche* meaning wise and *weik* meaning to bend, weave and wind. Who better than a yogi to weave and bend? We yoga teachers weave practices, show others how to tune into the wisdom of our bodies and hold space with our own special brand of magic!

I want to acknowledge here, that this book is about an ancient Hindu practice and I'm a white female who has no Indian heritage. By weaving it into my own heritage (Celtic, Norse and European) I hope that I am bringing in some of my own culture and trying to do so with the utmost respect for the roots of yoga. I want to honour and acknowledge where yoga has come from as well as sharing some of my knowledge and personal ideas, I hope I have managed this and conveyed my respect of yoga as a lifelong journey of study, awareness and humility.

The Call of the Witch...

You may well come across people who already consider you a witch if you have any interest in spiritual practices, whether that be yoga, meditation, oracle cards or aromatherapy. And yes, there will be people who think there is something wrong or bad about these things.

The term *witch* has come to mean many unpleasant things: someone cruel and vengeful, bitter and angry, a devil worshipper... These associations are so far from the work of the wise women and keepers of knowledge who were so often accused of being witches. Luckily, recent years have seen a reclaiming of the word *witch*, and it is once more coming to acknowledge witches' positive attributes, as powerful, intuitive beings, living in tune with the cycles of the year, moon, and nature. The world is slowly starting to recognise what us witches have always known.

Witches were once wise women, herbalists, midwives and oracles, called upon for healing, divination and advice. Over centuries witches and wise women were condemned and scapegoated by many religious groups. The Church, in its quest for power and dominance, created its own mythology about witches and their worship of the devil. To be a witch (and therefore dangerous in the eyes of the Church) is to acknowledge the sacred within us, here in our own bodies and the living earth, the connection we all have to the divine. To the witch, or any woman in tune with the natural world, everything is part of a cycle, which is in contrast to much religious doctrine that suggests that something and someone else holds the power, and you must be subservient, waiting for a final 'judgement day'. The Church has, and in some cases still does, sought to subdue and cast out anyone who claimed their own power: many powerful women and witches have paid a great price for their own empowerment.

Witches pop up a few times in the Bible as references (not particularly positive) to fortune-tellers, soothsayers, charmers, diviners, casters of spells, and those "who consult ghosts and spirits or seek oracles from the dead". But the obsession with them started in Europe in the Middle Ages. The first books to focus solely on witches also did not show them in a good light and presented many biased stereotypes. The most infamous book, the *Malleus Maleficarum* (1486), vividly described the satanic and sexual 'abominations' of witches. This was no doubt very useful in fuelling the ongoing idea that witches were seductresses with mind-control powers and supporting the cause of so-called 'Witch Hunters' and their cruel crusade to exterminate witches. At least ten years previous to that more well-known volume, the *Fortalitium Fidei* and *Formicarius* were some of the first texts to be explicitly published on witchcraft. In *Formicarius*, the witch is described as more commonly a woman, this idea that the 'magician' was female was shocking to some, as many, including the author, considered them inferior physically, mentally and morally.

The periods of witch hunts (around 1500 to 1700) in Europe, were spurred on by such texts. And it was predominantly free-thinking, independent and knowledgeable women that suffered persecution for their work with herbs, healing, astrology, divination, and midwifery. All these became indelibly associated in the Western mind with witchcraft, and have remained so ever since.

In 1542 the first laws against witchcraft in England appeared with Henry VIII. Under subsequent monarchs, the rules were regularly repealed, restored and altered – and show how hard a time people had defining precisely what it was they were outlawing. With Henry VIII "enchauntementes or sorceries" to find buried treasure were outlawed. In the reign of Elizabeth I "An Act Against Conjurations, Enchantments and Witchcrafts" was passed, and the death penalty incurred where harm had been caused by the alleged witch. At around this time accusations for "death caused by witchcraft" begin to appear in the historical record. Of the 1,158 murder victims identified in the surviving records, 228 were suspected killed by witchcraft. In comparison, poison was suspected in just 31 of the cases! I'm guessing that witchcraft was a great way to rationalise unexplainable deaths. (Further facts and figures can be found in *Witchcraft and Society in England and America, 1550–1750* by Marion Gibson.)

These laws were exported and had a hand in the building of the 'New World' too. In 1692, when the Salem witch trials took place, Massachusetts was a British colony, and therefore fell under these same British rules and laws.

But then in a complete turnaround, The Witchcraft Act of 1735 was passed in Great Britain which made it a crime for anyone to claim that a person had magical powers or was guilty of practising witchcraft. With this, witchcraft was no longer considered a criminal act, so the law stopped the hunting and execution of witches. But, and it gets a bit confusing here, it was not the supposed *practice* of witchcraft but the superstitious *belief in its existence* that became the crime. What was really being sought was to eradicate the belief in witchcraft. So it was no longer possible to be prosecuted as a witch, but one could be prosecuted for 'pretending' to "use any kind of witchcraft, sorcery, enchantment, or conjuration, or undertake to tell fortunes". In 1951 that Witchcraft Act was repealed and replaced by the Fraudulent Mediums Act. It was replaced again in 2008 by the very sensible and proper sounding Consumer Protection Regulations, a long way from the debauched devilry of the 1400s; but as it no longer suggests burning, lynching or drowning, that's a good start. But at the time of writing this book, women and children are still being killed in India and Africa for 'being witches'. And at the same time, there are at least three popular TV series starring female witches who are empowered, strong, awesome and fun. People are both scared and enraptured at the possibility of witches and witchcraft.

This wending and winding path reflects well that no one really knew or knows how to define magic and witchcraft. Or perhaps that these laws were once purposefully made fuzzy to allow persecutions to be carried out with less explanation – probably a little of both. In our Western patriarchal world that likes to define everything logically with solid proof, powers such as magic and witchcraft cause great confusion: a power that half the world denies exists and the other half would happily see people hang for.

Modern-day witches can still struggle to shake their historical stereotypes and public understanding is still low as to what witchcraft really is. This, in part, stems from the diversity of practice amongst witches, and the level of secrecy many still feel they need to ensure.

All of us, it seems, hold memories, traditions and beliefs about witches that can shape our feelings about them. It has been fascinating to record some of the responses from people as I have shared what I am writing about. One student shared fondly with me the herbs and tinctures her grandmother used to soothe aches and pains. Another spoke excitedly about *muti*, the South African term for magic. My German friend told me of the witches that dance every year at the base of Mount Brocken for *Walpurgisnacht*. And a Romanian friend told me of the *lele* – fairies with magical powers that live in the forests and mountains of Romania.

What is Witchcraft?

Witchcraft is the doing of magic – the harnessing, utilising and putting into action of magic. Craft is something you do with your hands, mind, energy and intention. If you recite spells, blend herbs, meditate, manifest, practice divination, or do rituals you are doing witchcraft (if you wish to call it that, some people prefer to use other terms). Some witches work with angels, goddesses and fairy folk, some with herbs, spices and fruits. Some witches and magicians follow centuries-old traditions, and others – like chaos magicians – are eclectic and use only what works for them from different traditions and ditch what doesn't.

Witchcraft itself is not a religion – to be a witch allows freedom from religious rules. Whilst some practice Wicca – an organised religion, created in England in the twentieth century, based around witchcraft and ritual – many others do not. Witches can form a group or coven, or practice as a solitary witch. You can practice on your own in your own way, beholden to no rules but your own. You can be a witch and a Buddhist, a witch and a druid, and indeed a witch and a yogi.

Whatever their affiliations, most witches strive to live a peaceful, tolerant and harmonious life in tune with nature and humanity; there's seldom anything sinister about it. It's more likely to be a herbal remedy to heal, than a curse to cause harm. While it is, of course, possible that some witches attempt to use witchcraft for harmful purposes, most have embraced it for healing or protection against the evil they themselves can be accused of.

Witches are myths, mothers, healers, crafters, sisters and sirens. Witches are real. Witches are both everything people fear and none of it. Witches represent power and possibility.

Witch, much like woman, is a word that can all at once be a proudly claimed title, an endearment and a damning (and even deadly) insult. Only the most potent and loaded words can divide people so fiercely. The titles we gather through life are so fascinating: mother, wife, aunt, sister, daughter…are all bestowed by society according to our relationships and standing with others. But what of those we wish to claim for ourselves, even secretly? Within the word 'witch', such power is held, both in its possibilities of skills and the vast and varied history of the word.

A witch is someone who seeks and finds connection. She acknowledges the cycles of the earth and universe and her place within them. She learns how to use energy within herself and the world to make changes. She seeks to make the earth a better place for herself and for others.

To call yourself a witch, priestess or goddess needs no documentation, no exam to pass, no one need be consulted. You can just claim it, right here and right now…should you wish. Maybe you prefer the word healer, oracle, creatrix, yogi or wise woman. You can claim those too! What if we consciously created ourselves precisely as we wanted to be? Instead of passively receiving the titles assigned to us through life. Wouldn't that be amazing!? Of course, you can call yourself whatever you please, it may even change from day to day. You do not have to justify who you are to anyone.

When we embrace the witch within, even privately, we enhance our natural magical abilities, heal our wellbeing on all levels and thrive in this very modern world, in balance and harmony – with a sprinkle of pure magic.

On Yoga

To those new to it, the word *yoga* is the Sanskrit word for yoke, unite or join together.

Yoga has many different branches, grown from many roots of Hindu spiritual practice. It originated in the Indus Valley, an area that today encompasses parts of north-east Afghanistan, Pakistan and north-west India. This culture flourished from 3300 to 1300BCE and along with ancient Egypt and Mesopotamia, was one of three early civilisations that make up what we know as the Old World.

From this time we begin to see ancient texts from the Indus cultures including the *Vedas, Upanishads,* and the *Bhagavad Gita* all start to mention a special introspective and meditative practice that we would come to call yoga.

The primary forms of yoga, first appear in the *Bhagavad Gita*: Karma yoga (the yoga of altruistic action); Bhakti yoga (of love and devotion); Jnana yoga (of self-study and knowledge). Later came Raja yoga (Royal or King yoga for self-mastery). In Sanskrit texts, Raja yoga was both the goal of yoga and a method of attaining it. Raja yoga is most often associated with the *Yoga Sutras,* which was the first 'instructional manual' for yoga created by Patanjali.

Patanjali's Eight Limbs of Yoga

The *Yoga Sutras of Patanjali* are the foundation texts that lay out the instructions for achieving union via yogic practices as we know them today. It comprised of eight different limbs: *yama, niyama, asana, pranayama, pratyahara, dharana, dhyana* and *samadhi.*

The *yamas* and *niyamas* are ethical guidelines laid out in the first two limbs of the eightfold path. *Yamas* are actions not to do, or restraints, *niyamas* are things to do or rituals. Together, they form a sort of code of conduct.

1. *Yamas* (restraints)

    ☾ *Ahimsa* (compassion for all living things/non-harming)

    ☾ *Satya* (truthfulness)

    ☾ *Asteya (Non-stealing)*

    ☾ *Brahmacharya* (energy control/moderation)

    ☾ *Aparigraha* (non-greed)

2. *Niyamas* (rituals)

   ☾ *Sauca* (cleanliness)

   ☾ *Santosa* (contentment)

   ☾ *Tapas* (disciplined use of energy)

   ☾ *Svadhyaya* (self-study/self-reflective awareness)

   ☾ *Isvarpranidhana* (celebration of the spiritual)

3. *Asana* (body postures)

Most people today connect the word *yoga* solely with *asana*. Whilst the various asana have beneficial physiological effects and help you relax and concentrate on your breath, their traditional goal is as strengthening exercises that prepare the physical body to sit in meditation for hours at a time.

4. *Pranayama* (breath control)

Pranayama are breathing techniques that prepare your mind and body for meditation.

5. *Pratyahara* (control of the senses)

This refers to the ability to quiet the mind and prepare for meditative concentration. Many yoga teachers, including myself, use the term "monkey mind" for when we have thoughts that keep jumping around in our heads, intruding on our concentration. We strive to quiet the mind, withdraw the senses and learn not to be distracted by the monkeys...

6. *Dharana* (concentration and stilling of the mind)

This is a practice used to find a single focus. Similar to our more modern words of flow and mindfulness. This step prepares one to begin the practice of *dhyana*.

7. *Dhyana* (consciousness of being)

A place of meditation with no focal point and unbroken awareness.

And finally:

8. *Samadhi* (union with the divine)

Also known as *nirvana* or bliss, this complete harmony is the ultimate goal of the yoga journey, a state of transcending time and space.

What Patanjali called *chitta vritti nirodhah* – the removal of the fluctuations of body and mind – is the ultimate purpose of yoga. Yoga is the stilling of the mind to a state of absolute calm, like the tranquil water of a millpond. These clear, calm waters we seek to create, give us a clarity through which we may see and experience life, uncoloured by opinions of good or bad. When the fluctuations settle, we experience oneness and union with all, whatever that means to us: Goddess, God, Spirit, Energy of the Universe, Mother Earth…

☾ *Yoga* = to yoke, to join, to unite

☾ *Chitta* = consciousness

☾ *Vritti* = fluctuations

☾ *Nirodhah* = quieting of

As I say to my students, we may well never reach perfection at this art, but that's why we call it yoga *practice*: all we can ever do is come back and try again, keep learning, keep growing.

So if you were to take just one thing away from this little outline, it would be this: that picture of that very flexible bikini-clad model on the beach? That's not yoga. Those elaborate balances on Norwegian clifftops...not yoga. They are just asana. They are stepping stones on the journey. There is so much more going on in yoga than just what you see. It is these asana *combined* with all the other limbs: meditation, pranayama etc. that are ways to get us to the union that *is* yoga. So never be concerned that you need to look a certain way, or be strong/flexible/coordinated to practice yoga. You can practice yoga with some simple breathing on a bus, or mindful movement at your desk. It's not just the 'pose', it's the intention that matters.

Combining Yoga and Witchcraft: How and Why

I am hoping that you are beginning to see how witchcraft and yoga could be naturally complimentary. There is similarity in many of the various practices, and those who do practice both and find them mutually supportive.

The primary goal of yoga is to quieten the body and mind which creates a state perfect from which to practice ritual, visualisation, mantra, prayer or anything you wish to give your full attention. Yoga can be appropriate for any spiritual practice or religion. At the very least, it can help you keep your mind on what you're doing, and quieten the distraction as you practice your magic – whatever form that may take. And most witches practice similar energetic work to yoga: developing higher consciousness in forms such as meditation, divination and trance. Why not consciously and purposefully combine the two?

This book is a process of journeying, discovery and movement. I certainly don't have all the answers, and I don't yet know how the pieces all fit together, that's all part of the adventure. My intention for *Yoga for Witches* is to share with you what I have discovered so far, about how these two practices can combine. Yoga and witchcraft share an element of surrendering to the process, to the flow. And it is through that flow that we may discover a little more of who we are. So maybe we'll let go of that need for the right answers and exact rules and embrace the divine feminine work of intuition, feeling and compassion. And just see where the path may lead...

Structure of the Book

Our journey starts by exploring the concept of magic and how it can be explored in your own body and daily life by using practices from witchcraft and yoga. The second half of the book explores the wider world of magic: the impact of the sun, moon, earth and seasons on ourselves and our practices.

Each chapter covers yoga and witchcraft both separately and together, sharing practical exercises and philosophical ideas. I have never been one for strict recipes, I never manage to follow them exactly...and it is the same with spells and rituals. Therefore, what you will find in this book are not precise step-by-step rules that must be followed to the letter, but rather more open-ended guidance and suggestions. It is useful to remember that every single spell and ritual was once created by a witch, and you can do the same. Just like every yoga sequence was once created by a yogi. The intention is everything. Follow your intuition. If you feel inspired to create a spell, then do it! If you like a spell or ritual you've created, note it down in your Book of Shadows (we'll explore this more in Chapter 6).

Each chapter finishes with a list of goddesses relevant to the topic. When I first started this book, I envisaged listing a few useful goddesses for the chapters on the sun, moon and earth, and leaving it at that. But I've found with each chapter, with each new journey into a facet of magic and spirit, more goddesses arise! Of course, I really should have known! The archetype of the Goddess is a magical glimmer of a past when we used elements of ourselves to create deities to make sense of the world. That instinct of myth and magic is still within us, so it's only right that with every chapter of yoga and magic we should have a few goddesses to watch over us! However, as with every goddess in this book, she has many faces, many elements, so do not feel these goddesses need be restrained within the chapters I have placed them – if you wish to channel Benzaiten to watch over your moon magic or draw on Áine to inspire your journal work, then, of course, you can do so!

Goddess – What, Why and How?

I'm including lots of lovely goddesses from cultures around the world. Great! But why and how are they useful for your journey?

I'm glad you asked! We may well be familiar with the odd goddess of myth and legend, and with some of the ancient civilisations that once believed these goddesses were responsible for such fabulous natural occurrences as drawing the moon across the night sky. Once, looking upon the marvels of the natural world, our ancestors used what they knew, to explain what they didn't. They drew images of beautiful women and imbued them with our strongest traits of courage, passion, power, wisdom and love. Now...well, now we know that it's not actually a divine goddess pulling the moon across the night sky. But there is still much we don't understand about how the universe works, and energies that can't always be explained by science and logic. The moon is still a powerful and beautiful force, and it doesn't mean it is not still very valuable and enjoyable to connect to both the moon's cycles and energy *and* practices and beliefs of our ancestors in connecting to this energy. What they believed was powerful as well. The goddess archetypes are created from elements of ourselves as humans, so when we connect to aspects of the Goddess – what we are really connecting to is elements of ourselves. Goddesses can provide information and inspirations; they can reinforce your ideas; they can provide comforts and encouragement. Sometimes the concept of a goddess can seem abstract, based in intuition and personal belief, inspiration and strengths. Or perhaps it is the energy you want to connect to just within yourself, no deities at all – just your own spirit, and the elements of the divine feminine within. There's no right or wrong. You can explore for yourself what the Goddess means to you, and how this idea may serve you.

Connecting with this idea of the Goddess as we understand Her can be your source of strength, healing, creativity, intuition, nurturing and wisdom. We may well have lost touch with these qualities as we have stifled our spirits to fit into a modern, noisy, busy, disconnected patriarchal world. Here are just a few practical ideas of how you may bring the Goddess into your thoughts or day in some way.

☾ Connect to a specific goddess in meditation: reflect on her strengths, and how she may deal with issues you are exploring.

☾ Pick a goddess for your day, and reflect on her attributes to inspire you – would Aphrodite take some time to relax? Would warrior goddess Diana share her honest thoughts at work? Absolutely! Allow the qualities of the goddess to help guide and inspire you.

☾ Bring a goddess icon or picture to your altar, or anywhere that might encourage you – she could sit at your desk or by your bed.

☾ Read aloud a myth or story of a goddess that you find inspiring and talk with your friends about it. What inspires you about the story?

☾ Spend a week 'working' with a goddess – find out about her stories, her culture, her strengths and weaknesses. You may find inspiration from this work, and excitement of feeling a connection to a goddess.

☾ Explore seasonal goddesses as a way to note and celebrate the changing of the seasons: flower maidens Bridie and Ostara for spring, and earthy goddesses Pachamama and Gaia for autumn perhaps.

Remembering What We Once Knew

My connection to witchcraft has allowed me to deepen my yogic practice. I can use asana to engage in ritual and to move in an inspired way. When leading group meditations and slow restorative classes, I draw on goddess myth and archetype. I use oracle cards to guide our themes and read poems about the moon. Many of the yoga retreats I run are based around the lunar calendar and moon goddesses. These connections allow me to create a sacred space, enabling the subtle energy present in our movement and our spells of intention to bring greater presence to the ritual of our class. It is this deepening of experience that I wish to share with you.

There is a Sanskrit word I love: *smarana*. It means to recall or uncover that which you once knew. Once, as children, we moved our bodies for the sheer joy of it. We rested, ate, laughed, sang, cried when we wanted to. We gazed at the sky, threw tantrums and hugged with abandon. Yoga can help us remember some of this. As can witchcraft, maybe even more so.

You aren't just remembering what you may have forgotten from your own life, but many lives before you. You are remembering the wisdom that the universe held long before you arrived: the ancient knowledge of the earth, seasons and planets. An understanding that was once unchallenged in its power. And then, somewhere along the line, was pushed aside as nonsense, woo-woo or evil.

The time has definitely come for *smarana*: to uncover, rediscover and reconnect with the realness of the universe – simple, powerful, infinite.

Everyone is Welcome Here

This path is open to us all. Every. Single. One of us. Despite their history, *yogi* and *witch* are both actually gender neutral terms. Once it was more often men who would practice yoga, and therefore some called women *yoginis*, to differentiate from the men who were known as *yogi* or *yogin*. Then, in the last century, things swung the other way entirely as women took over the yoga scene. Now, *yogi* simply means a practitioner of yoga. Whilst the term *witch* is commonly associated only with women, actually witches can be any gender, and during each country's own witch trials men also lost their lives.

Everyone is welcome here; whatever your gender or gender identity. This book is about connection. About finding your own magic and awesome power. And a lovely big splash of divine feminine energy that we can all connect to – the energy of love, compassion, power, fearlessness, and passion!

So, welcome human, whoever you are. I send you my love and gratitude for joining me on this journey.

Blessed Be!

Namaste, witches x

IN SEARCH OF MAGIC

We spoke about the word *witch* in the introduction, and how divisive it can be. In comparison, *magic* is a much more popular word in mainstream culture. When we fall in love, *it's magic*. When something fantastic happens to us, *it's like magic!* When we have a good time, *it was so magical*…so why and how have we created this disconnect between witches, magic and witchcraft?

Like all powerful ideas, magic can both thrill and terrify us all at once. Hence the extreme reactions to witches and their work. We both covet and fear that kind of power.

Magic has existed in some form in all cultures. Spells have been found carved on writing tablets from ancient Mesopotamia and in early Babylonian texts. Egyptian *heka* magic was recorded on papyrus and in carvings and hundreds of spells featured in Egyptian books of the dead (guides on passing into the afterlife). Magic has existed since ancient times, and so too have sorcerers, wise women, shamans, oracles and witches that made magic and worked in service to others. These people usually held respect, power and influence within their societies. But through the ages rumours, mysteries, stereotypes and prejudices have grown up around what each of these wranglers of magic could do. Tales told in whispers spoke of covens of men and women meeting at midnight, consorting with the devil, dancing naked and taking flight.

Magic and witchcraft remind us that not everything in this world is definable, concrete or absolute. Whether you believe or not, we have always lived in a world fascinated by the promises that magic holds. Once the layers of fear and disconnection are pulled away, magic is an invitation into a space of possibility, freedom and power.

Magic is something real, it can go by any name you choose. At times we forget or find it hard to imagine that there is light and power when we feel cold and dark. But when you feel like this, look to what's endured for many centuries, before you and your magic came to be. Before cars, streets, cathedrals and temples there were trees and plants, and there were mountains. There was the sun in the sky and the moon amongst the stars. There were seasons, rolling through their cycles. We are part of this awesome magic of the earth.

Defining the Indefinable

The etymological roots of the word magic as we use it today come from many varied threads. Potentially including magush, *an ancient Persian word that means 'to have power', 'to be able' and the Greek* magike *meaning magical and* magos *meaning members of a learned and priestly class.*

The words *magic* and *magical* are in some ways, indefinable, although we still try. Some of the most well-used definitions are…

☾ Relating to, using, or resembling magic.

☾ Beautiful in a way that seems separate from everyday life.

☾ Extraordinary energy or influence from a supernatural source.

☾ Something that appears to cast a spell or enchantment.

☾ The science and art of causing change in conformity with one's will.

You'll note that descriptors are often defined as something that 'resembles' magic or 'as if by magic'. Whether something is considered magic or something 'like' magic is all in the interpretation, another reason why defining magic is so hard! As so often is the case, viewpoint is everything: When Roman naturalist Pliny the elder (23–79AD) dismissed magic as the fraudulent work of 'fools and foreigners', he also warned that menstruating women should be avoided by men as their dark magic would cause the fruit to fall from trees and metal to rust. (Both musings can be found in Pliny's *Naturalis Historia*).

Magic, like many words (spirituality, is another example I often use in my classes) means very different things to different people. Magic can mean power, strength, a spark of love or excitement, a state of flow, or a warm feeling of contentment or unity. I invite you within this book, whether you are a witch, yogi, or both or anything in between, to find your own connections to the word. And hopefully you will connect to magic in your own way. Some of you may already know the Wiccan Rede "An' ye harm none, do what ye will."* In yoga we may recognise this as *ahimsa*. In all cultures, it equates to something similar: work towards finding your path and be kind. And try to accept and understand that everyone's path will be different.

On Magic and Witchcraft

All beings are able to create and connect to magic – whether it be via witchcraft, love, gratitude, kindness, spiritual practices such as yoga, or it might be something that you stumble upon and experience in your day-to-day travels through life, like a beautiful sunset or a deer that pauses to look you in the eyes. This is why some prefer to separate magic and witchcraft. Whereas others would say any production of magic is a kind of witchcraft, or that witchcraft does not always produce magic. And sometimes magic appears all on its own.

Witchcraft tends to be regarded as one of many forms of utilising, controlling and creating magic. When looking at witchcraft, we explore something you can control yourself – controlling and inviting magic into your life. You do not need to be a witch to experience, generate and appreciate magic. But should you wish to invite more magic into your life, witchcraft is a tool you can use.

Although most modern magical writers have suggested that the primary purpose of magic is to change the practitioner, rather than the external world, but I think one can easily lead to the other. Change can be produced in the surrounding reality directly or as a result of the change in awareness of the practitioner, who is now empowered to go out and make change in some way.

---

* I mention the Wiccan Rede here, but to be clear, this book will explore witchcraft rather than Wicca.

Losing and Reclaiming Power

Somewhere along the journey of humans through time, religion, culture, critics of magic and the patriarchy have convinced us to have less faith in nature and our own intuition. They have dismissed these ways of knowing and being as devilish, foolish or pointless. Through this disconnection from the natural world, women and witches have been forcibly separated from their power: pulled away from their herbs, separated from their own intuition about their bodies and even the planet. We, as women and as witches, have been separated from our power by the fear and fury of Church, patriarchy and even other people in our communities. Centuries of separation and fear, and every sort of 'witch hunt' has separated us from our awareness, our natural ability to connect to time, environment and the souls around us. We may have become so detached from our natural, simple intuition and abilities that it can all seem like weird and incredible magic. When all we are really doing is connecting to nature and our own power.

It's time to reclaim witchcraft. It's time to reclaim the witch. And I believe yoga can help.

The Siddhis - Yoga Magic

Yogis have long been journeying into finding what we may call magic. One of my favourite parts of the *Yoga Sutras* are the references to *siddhis*. Siddhi can be translated as accomplishment, attainment, or success. And may apparently be attained through birth, the use of herbs, incantations, self-discipline, dedicated practice of yoga asana, and/or *samadhi*. These powers include abilities such as clairvoyance, telepathy, levitation, invulnerability, and access to past life memories.

However, these powers are not regarded in the yogic texts as magical: they're actually considered ordinary capacities that everyone possesses. We've just become too disconnected from our own abilities to access them. What one may call magic, another may just see as wonderful innate human ability.

Patanjali explains that the siddhis are attained after mastery of the last three steps of his Eightfold Path (concentration, consciousness and union with the divine), known as *samyama* when combined, which means 'holding together'.

Various siddhis can arise depending on the object of focus. If one focuses on another person, the siddhi that occurs is what we might call telepathy, as your mind breaks through the illusion of separation between you and the other person.

There are many siddhis listed in the *Yoga Sutras*, and these abilities may be interpreted in different ways. Below I share some of my favourites, not only because they are fascinating in themselves, but also because they mirror what we have in other cultures called magic and witchcraft. How lovely they are, not fearsome, evil or scary but rather the result of the dedication to bettering oneself, to finding joy, and relief from dis-ease.

Loving-kindness to all resulting from *samyama* on empathy, joy and compassion. This could be understood to mean that when one is filled with joy, that state may induce similar feelings in others. I love that this is outlined as a great power, because we may all struggle with loving-kindness and its importance to ourselves and others cannot be underestimated to overall wellbeing. (You will learn about the Loving-Kindness Meditation in Chapter 13.)

Exceptional strength resulting from *samyama* focus on physical strength, but it might also include mental or spiritual power. We are, all of us, capable of great things, possibly more than we realise. Meditation on our strengths may well help us connect to our own inner strength and remember that we are all-powerful beings.

Exceptional health through *samyama* on the solar plexus chakra. This siddhi refers to knowledge of the self, leading to excellent health or self-healing. In modern scientific study we are learning more all the time about the power of the mind to heal us.

Levitation through a focus on the sense of lightness. This siddhi causes the yogi to float, hover or fly (I wonder if brooms were ever considered…) It could be interpreted as a form of psychokinesis. Or a witchy interpretation may well be astral projection or a feeling of leaving one's body.

Blazing radiance through *samyama* on internal energy or inner power. This could be interpreted in several ways, as possession of exceptional charisma or a fierce sense of self. After all, what is more radiant than a woman connected to her power?

The siddhis were also categorised through the chakra system (we'll explore chakras more in Chapter 2.) Meditation or focused intention with one chakra could bring certain siddhis. For example, by contemplating on the third eye chakra, the siddhi one attains "the highest success" – which may well refer to knowledge and enlightenment.

Patanjali did also stress the dangers of dwelling on the siddhis, saying one should avoid pressure to display or grasp at accomplishments in yoga, including the siddhis, because this can lead to arrogance and ego, and this can block further spiritual growth. This sounds very relevant to the world of witchcraft, and really, all society. When you say that you are *something* – a goddess, witch, priestess, yogi – someone may well respond: "prove it". It is a challenge to resist explaining oneself in some way. Your proof is within. This is not about 'Truth', only your truth, and your experiences.

If you would like to read more about the siddhis and how we can harness the idea of this power specifically in line with our divine feminine and witchy selves, I cannot recommend highly enough *Yoni Shakti* by Uma Dinsmore-Tuli. What she has done is create a practice of yoga exploring the divine feminine with siddhis and wisdom goddesses, encouraging conscious connection to our own inner power as women. Though the stories of the siddhis from Patanjali are available to us all, Uma has woven new siddhis specially for women and all the power that dwells within us.

Finding Your Own Magic

So, is magic simply the reconnection to our intuition and the rhythm of the planet, a remembrance of our own inner power...or is it more than that? Is there a power of the universe to which we can connect to grow our own power? Can we capture magic or create our own? Can we return to who we were before we were told what to be? Before an empowered woman was painted as evil and witches were cursed as devils. Can we return to our power and our intuition? Can we trust in our own intuition, and in the power of the natural world?

This is a journey you must explore yourself and answer the questions in your own way.

Use of magic and witchcraft, like yoga, is a personal pursuit you can tailor for your own goals. Do you want to be a Kitchen Witch with an inviting home full of dried herbs and warming foods? Do you wish to connect to the messages and meanings of the spirit world? Do you want to hone your skills in intuition or to connect to the cycles of the earth, seasons and moon? Do you want to paint animal guides by candlelight, and tend plants like family? Magic need not have one purpose or one 'right way'. You can create your own unique blend of magic, your own place in the vast field of spirituality that feels right. For me, teaching yoga in a way that can allow students to release and heal, mixing essential oil blends, honouring the lunar and seasonal cycles and using oracle cards for work with goddesses is my practice. Rituals and spells, when I do them, are very simple and usually sometimes no more than lighting a candle with intention.

Finding your magical path may well involve much study, trial-and-error learning, intuition, humility, constant adaptation and evolution, devotion to your own integrity, and learning to let go. But doing so, you can create a spiritual practice all of your own.

Closing Thoughts

I am reminded of a story told to me by one of my goddess teachers. She went to Stonehenge for the summer solstice and…she did not enjoy it! Anyone who has been in recent years may find themselves distracted from the magical beauty of the rising sun by people revelling in drugs, drink and trance music. (I'm not against these things, but they can distract from the quieter, natural element of the moment). Before sunrise, she found herself a corner to meditate, and was approached by a man with a beer in his hand. He said in a somewhat mocking tone, "So, you believe in all this stuff, do you?"

To which she replied, "Do I believe that the sun will rise? Yes, yes I do."

The sun rising every morning is pretty amazing and magical, and hopefully we all take time to be grateful that it does. But many people will never see it as something that is magical. So, whether magic exists or lies entirely in your own mind, connection to magic is available to everyone: the power is already within us. Just as no one needs to be trained to turn towards the light of the morning sun, we do it naturally if we allow ourselves to, like sunflowers. If you find joy in connection to any magic, or whatever word you wish to use, enjoy it!

ENERGY MAGIC

W hat we are doing in yoga and in witching crafts is connecting to our inner power in our own depths and learning to harness the energies around us too. The energies that flow within and around the body affect us in physical, emotional and spiritual ways. This energy is often referred to as *chi* in Chinese traditions and *prana* in Indian traditions. As a witch, you may call this energy magic.

Energy Magic in Yoga

Within the yogic tradition, energy is understood to be regulated in the body through the chakra system. The foundation of chakra theory is that we are more than just our physical body. We have a body that is made up of three parts: physical, subtle and natural. Our physical body includes our limbs and organs, our blood and bones. The subtle body (also called the energy body) encompasses our mind and intellect, emotional and spiritual personalities. And the natural body is our innate desires and the inherent nature of who we are. The subtle body is connected to our energy at the deepest instinctual level.

Chakra means "wheel" or "turning", and they are represented as gateways into the body through which subtle energy flows or is lost. Chakras are often visualised as wheels that turn within a healthy body or as flowers that open to reveal balanced energy. At each chakra point you'll find important glands and organs. They are points at which the subtle and physical bodies are connected.

The first four chakras are considered to belong to the physical body, the top three are of spirit, ether and universe. The heart is the connection between the realms of the physical and spiritual.

Chakras are focal points for meditation within the human body, located where we experience emotional and spiritual energy. When energy flows through the chakras all is well. But blockages can lead to disease. Chakras can become blocked through emotional upset: conflict, loss, fear, anxiety and stress are all common causes of chakra imbalance.

Energy Channels

The chakras are linked by energy channels called nadi *that carry* prana *(life force) through the body. The chakras, like shining beads on a necklace, run along the central energy line, which is called the* sushumna nadi. *Two intertwining channels that loop around this nadi, are called the* ida *and* pingala. *Ida on the left carries descending energy, and pingala on the right carries ascending energy. They bring energy into the central sushumna nadi, and where these three lines of energy cross, we find our chakras!*

A chakra is considered, in an energetic sense, imbalanced, if it is either over-stimulated or under-stimulated. Exploring this chakra 'imbalance' offers a way of exploring and recognising dis-ease within your body. For example, if you find yourself unable to speak up in a meeting, is this a physical issue? Do you have a sore throat that is stopping you speaking? No? Then you may want to explore what is causing your inability to speak up from the idea of the throat chakra being under-stimulated or blocked. Are you unsure of yourself? Has your confidence recently taken a knock? Or could you benefit from focus on this area with activities to stimulate the throat chakra like chanting, meditation or talking to someone?

In contrast, what we would call an overactive throat chakra may cause you to speak before you think, or to say hurtful, careless things, which may be caused by underlying feelings of anger. If you cannot connect to your imagination or intuition one may say you have an underactive third eye chakra. Whereas if you are plagued with nightmares, it may be overactive (and indicative of causes such as stress or trauma). The imbalance of the chakras is not the cause of the issue, but a symptom; these imbalances can be soothed using methods including yoga, meditation, spell work and ritual.

Kundalini and the Chakras

Kundalini refers to a form of primal energy that is located at the base of the spine. This energy can be represented as a snake or sometimes a goddess. Kundalini energy rises up from the *muladhara* chakra, along the *sushumna nadi* through each chakra in turn. As this energy rises the practitioner becomes enlightened, experiencing a profound transformation of consciousness.

Kundalini energy can be awakened through work with Hatha yoga, pranayama, mudras, mantras and visualisation (we'll learn more about these in later chapters).

Kundalini yoga is a fusion of Hindu and Sikh cultural and spiritual ideas: focusing on your own power and energy as your own guru. Through the practice of Kundalini yoga, we can forge strong connections to our energetic centres and chakras. Kundalini yoga practices use two lovely mantras:

ong namo guru dev namo
"I bow to the Divine Wisdom within myself"

As well as the call to the divine teacher within to guide us:

sat nam
"I am truth"

Sat nam is known as a *bija* (seed) mantra – a sound that can activate the chakras. "It is small and potent. Great things grow from it," said Yogi Bhajan, who brought Kundalini yoga to the United States in 1968.

A Powerful Practice

Just a heads up for those of you new to it, Kundalini yoga can bring out an intense emotional response, and it may feel overwhelming, so do treat the practice, and yourself with care. For me, I almost always end up laughing, but I'm not sure how much of that is emotional release and how much is because I never manage to get all the words of the chants quite right! If you want to try Kundalini yoga please do seek out an experienced teacher, who will help guide you safely through your subtle body! I don't like to suggest that working with your own body and energy is dangerous, but I do advise caution; anyone with anxiety or other mental health conditions should seek out a teacher and work gently into their Kundalini practice, so as to not trigger or overwhelm.

Chakras Beyond Yoga

Chakras were first described by the yogic tradition of ancient India, as well as in ancient Chinese and Buddhist cultures. But you'll also find tales of the chakras in myth, legend and in magic lore from around the world.

Many Western magical traditions, including some witchcraft traditions, have adopted the chakra system into their practice, incorporating the idea of opening and closing of the chakras into ritual, to ground and centre, and to protect against negative energy. Healing and strengthening energy can be found by combining chakra wisdom with beautiful witchy practices such as herbalism, candle magic and crystal work (see the table of correspondence below).

You'll often see each chakra portrayed in beautiful colours and light, and in the form of lotus flowers. Assigning colours to the chakras and lotus imagery is likely a relatively modern development as practitioners such as Carl Jung developed the chakra system for Westerners.

The idea of chakras is now so far-reaching and has collected so many new ideas, so intertwined, that unravelling may be impossible (as well as unnecessary) I suggest that you take what works for you and leave what doesn't.

Every book on the chakras presents a possible model, and you'll find different ideas in all of them, with many additions brought in from a huge range of modalities. Here, I'll outline each of the chakras and their qualities – as you take note of the mental and emotional effects of each chakra, it's very possible some will resonate with you. In understanding the areas each chakra governs we may be able to identify areas of our subtle body that need some attention. The chakras offer an outline for energetic exploration and self-enquiry, which is a wonderful start to a journey towards balance and healing. This is not an immediate solution, the wheels of chakras don't swing open and close instantly, just like healing and coming back to balance from physical injury or illness – give yourself time.

Correspondences

Correspondences are elements, seasons and beings with symbolic connections in the natural and magical world. Tables of correspondence help us connect and group together elements for spell and ritual work. For example, the moon corresponds to colours of silver and white, and nocturnal animals such as bats and moths.

Correspondence can help us find connections for use in spells, ritual or practice.

You can use existing correspondence from books – including this one – or create your own.

The Root Chakra

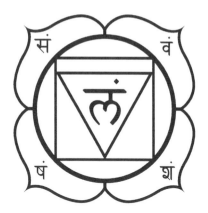

In Sanskrit: *Muladhara*, 'root support/foundation'.

Location: Base of the spine.

Colour: Red.

Flower: Lotus flower with four petals, triangular in shape.

Element: Earth.

Physical: Associated with feet, sacrum, spine, and ovaries/testes.

Mental and Emotional: Provides a sense of stability, security, and self-esteem. Lack of self-confidence can result from an underactive root chakra.

Seed Mantra: *Lam*.

My roots support me,
I am grounded,
I am safe.

The Sacral Chakra

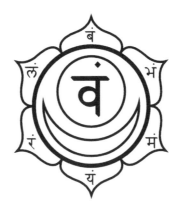

In Sanskrit: *Svadhishthana*, 'home of self'.

Location: Lower belly (below the navel).

Colour: Orange.

Flower: Six-petaled lotus.

Element: Water.

Physical: Associated with the organs of the reproductive and urinary system, and adrenal glands. In women, this is the source of our 'flow' both physically in menstruation and our creative flow.

Mental and Emotional: Drives creativity and joy. When underactive in this chakra, one may feel unenthusiastic and uninspired.

Seed Mantra: *Vam.*

I connect to the flow of life.

The Solar Plexus Chakra

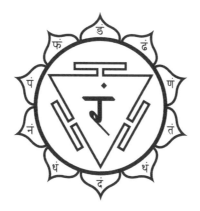

In Sanskrit: *Manipura*, 'city of jewels'.

Location: Between the navel and the sternum.

Colour: Yellow.

Flower: Ten-petaled lotus.

Element: Fire.

Physical: This chakra is related to the stomach, liver and pancreas.

Mental and Emotional: Related to energy, enthusiasm and determination. This chakra gives us a personal drive for daily tasks and self-empowerment to reach goals. An overactive solar plexus chakra can cause anger and aggressiveness. When in balance, it can help us feel empowered.

Seed Mantra: *Ram.*

I am peaceful,
I am powerful,
I shine.

The Heart Chakra

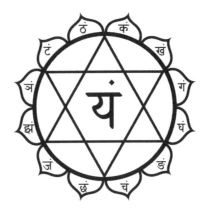

In Sanskrit: *Anahata*, 'the unstruck note, unbeaten.'

Location: Centre of the chest, heart space.

Colour: Green.

Flower: Twelve-petaled lotus. Featuring two triangles, one pointing up, the other down. This symbolises the joining of the physical and subtle body at the heart.

Element: Air.

Physical: Heart, lungs, circulatory system and thymus gland.

Mental and Emotional: A balanced heart chakra allows us to express love, compassion for others, and peace with oneself. The opening of our hearts to others is the best healing exercise for the heart chakra.

Seed Mantra: *Yam.*

I attune to the frequency of love.

The Throat Chakra

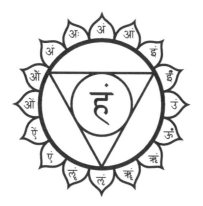

In Sanskrit: *Vishuddha*, 'pure'.

Location: Base of the neck, where the collar bones meet.

Colour: Turquoise.

Flower: Sixteen-petaled lotus.

Element: Ether.

Physical: Associated with the throat, ears, mouth and thyroid gland.

Mental and emotional: Relates to communication, expression, wisdom and truthfulness. An underactive or blocked throat chakra can lead to frustration and depression, as we may feel unheard, unacknowledged or unable to speak our truth.

Seed Mantra: *Ham.*

I connect to my truth.

The Third Eye Chakra

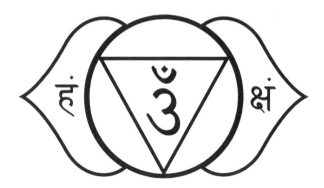

In Sanskrit: *Ajna*, 'command/ authority'.

Location: Between the eyebrows.

Colour: Deep blue.

Flower: Lotus with two petals.

Element: Spirit.

Physical: Relates to the pineal and pituitary glands, and hypothalamus.

Mental and emotional: Concentration, clarity, wisdom, imagination and insight. Affects our ability of having perspective on life and viewing past experiences.

Seed Mantra: *Om*.

My mind is open,
I expand my awareness.

The Crown Chakra

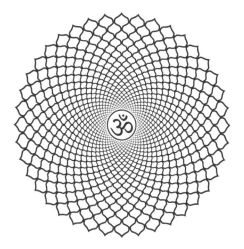

In Sanskrit: *Sahasrara*, 'thousand-petaled'.

Location: Top of the head.

Colour: Violet.

Flower: The thousand-petaled lotus, a symbol of spiritual illumination.

Element: Spirit.

Physical: The brain, cerebral cortex and central nervous system.

Mental and Emotional: Considered the connection to universal consciousness/Universe/Spirit. It influences spiritual will and idealism. Considered the key to releasing ego-driven, earth-bound desires to establish a union with your higher self.

Seed Mantra: *Om.*

*I am connected to the energy
of the universe.*

Correspondence Table:
Healing the Chakras

It may be that the list of chakras has illuminated something you may be working with right now – perhaps you really identify with the throat chakra if you feel unheard in your family, or the heart chakra if you are dealing with grief or loss. This correspondence table outlines just some of the elements connected to each chakra – in addition to our focus of attention and meditation – which is an excellent start.

If you want to work more deeply with a chakra, or simply explore some of the options, take a look at the list. For example, you may have related to the idea of the root chakra if you are currently feeling unstable and insecure, so you may first try some grounding meditation, and then maybe carry a carnelian stone in your pocket, use grounding oils and create a comforting root vegetable stew.

To focus on a chakra is to bring your awareness and intention to your energetic body, exploring how you connect in your own way. You will need to do some exploration as to how best to deal with what you may uncover. Each idea is part of a toolbox that can help. You can put together what works best for you.

Chakra	Yoga Asana	Essential Oils	Herbs	Calming Crystals	Healing Foods
Root	Mountain Pose	Patchouli, myrrh, cedarwood, vetiver	Dandelion root, sage, ginger	Carnelian	Apples and root vegetables
Sacral	Goddess Pose	Sandalwood, orange	Calendula flowers, hibiscus	Amber	Oranges, mandarins, nuts
Solar	Crescent Lunge	Juniper, lemon	Lemongrass, fennel, cinnamon	Citrine	Corn and cereals
Heart	Reclining Goddess Pose	Rose, neroli	Roses	Rose quartz, emerald, peridot	Leafy vegetables, spinach, green tea
Throat	Fish Pose	Lavender, rosemary	Lemon balm, eucalyptus	Turquoise	Nourishing liquids: juices, soups, teas
Brow	Child's Pose	Frankincense, basil	Passionflower mint	Lapis lazuli	Grapes, blueberries, chocolate, spices
Crown	Easy Seat	Jasmine	Lavender, lotus root	Amethyst	Time in the natural world and connection to the universe

Beyond the Seven Chakras

As well as the seven major chakras, there are over a hundred more recorded chakras in the human body, and various 'transpersonal' and 'subpersonal' chakras (energy centres in the space around you) some of which include:

- (*Soul Star Chakra: very closely linked with the crown chakra – just a little further above your head.*
- (*Earth Star Chakra: in the earth beneath your feet.*

And then, once you've gone past the body and space around you, there is a theory that the whole earth has chakras.

- (*The heart chakra is in Glastonbury/Avalon in the UK.*
- (*The throat chakra is at Mount Fuji, Japan.*
- (*The solar plexus is Uluru, Australia.*

What an amazing inspiration for a round-the-world trip!

Chakra Goddesses

The first two goddesses below are directly connected to Hindu mythology and chakra lore. However, individual chakras could also be related to goddesses from other pantheons. For example, if you wanted to work specifically with the heart chakra, you may wish to call on goddesses of love and compassion such as Kuan Yin and Aphrodite.

Shakti (Hindu) Goddess of Power. Shakti is the concept and personification of divine feminine creative power, the animating force of the universe. Shakti energy resides (among other places) in the Muladhara chakra. And when awakening Kundalini energy you may also awaken your Shakti or Goddess energy.

Bhairavi (Hindu) Goddess of Kundalini. She also lives within the

Muladhara chakra and is possibly another incarnation of Shakti. The name Bhairavi means "awe-inspiring". Sometimes depicted as a queen sat upon a lotus flower but also as a fearsome goddess of fire. Bhairavi is also a title for a woman skilled in Kundalini yoga. So, one who has achieved the state of Bhairavi is fearless and powerful like the goddess herself.

Inanna (Sumerian) There is a myth of how the goddess Inanna sought to descend into the underworld. She had to pass through seven 'gateways' relinquishing an item of clothing or veil at each gate. These seven gateways represent the seven chakras that Inanna must journey down through in order to arrive, naked, in the underworld. The symbolic teaching of this story is that in order to travel deep within ourselves, we must shed in some way and peel off the layers that life has given us – years of stress, anxiety, pressure, expectations – in order to return to our roots (and the root chakra).

Closing Thoughts

In systems with ancient roots, the physical make-up of the body may not have been so obvious as it is to us now. However, practitioners could still identify essential areas of the body: each major chakra was placed at a centre of physical importance. The chakra system may be, in some ways, a much better method of connecting in a felt sense to energetic areas of the body we cannot see.

In a sense, it's easier to deal with issues of the physical body – if you cut your hand on a pair of scissors you can easily see the cause, the injury, and the solution – clean the cut, whack on a plaster and in seven days you are healed! Huzzah! But what if you are feeling a sense of doubt in your heart? Or a general sense of insecurity? What is the cause? How might you work towards healing? You need to explore your thoughts, feelings and energy to answer these questions; this is why healing the subtle body takes more time and involves more introspective work.

Bringing a deeper awareness of the flow of subtle energies in the body plays a huge part in overall health as well. Our physical body thrives when energy can flow freely through it. When energy is blocked, such as in cases of stress or trauma, we can become unbalanced, unable to process thoughts and emotions, and more likely to encounter illness and disease. This is a really good example of *smarana* – remembering. We most likely knew already that holding onto emotion and excess stress are detrimental to health. But sometimes we need a reminder and a way to release. You can use the chakra system to help bring awareness and intention to where you may feel blocked, to focus your energy for positive change. Working through our blocks may well help us to ignite our inner fire, in the full rainbow spectrum of the chakras.

GROUNDING

To many practising witches and yogis, grounding is considered a vital part of learning to work with energy safely and sustainably. As with all things, it's all about balance. Grounding is a method of balancing and equalising the flow of energy. An ungrounded state is a scattered, unfocused state. Someone in an ungrounded state may be moody, feel on edge, unable to concentrate, distracted or disconnected. In contrast, a well-grounded person is settled and focused in mind and body. Some of us are better at achieving a grounded state than others. Learning how to ground can bring strength and comfort to any activity, and is particularly useful in spiritual practices. As such, you'll see the term grounding or earthing in both witch and yoga texts.

Grounding is the process of connecting with and becoming aware of our physical body and its connection with the earth. In yoga, we practice barefoot to connect to the earth and find our grounding. The feet are the foundations for many yoga poses as we make a direct physical connection with the earth. A transferral of energy can take place between body and earth: sending negative or pent up energy into the earth, or drawing on its limitless natural energy to 'recharge'. As a daily meditative practice, grounding can help maintain health: physical, mental and emotional.

When we are stressed, in fight or flight mode, we hold tension in our upper body: we take short, sharp breaths, our heart pounds, jaw and fists tense…our body is literally preparing us to come off the ground in a quick dash in flight or to leap into battle. So when you feel stressed, you need to counter this with something grounding to calm and reconnect your body and mind.

Daily Practice

Grounding can be utilised in your day-to-day life to enhance focus and happiness and lessen anxiety. We can all benefit from adding a few moments of grounding into our daily practice. There are many ways of grounding yourself, some exploration will help you find the one that is most effective for you.

It may seem like such a simple thing. But how familiar does this sound: you rise in the morning, make yourself a cup of tea perhaps, shower, get dressed, go to work, maybe stop at the gym on the way home, have dinner, watch TV before retiring to bed. It's not unusual to go a whole day, week or month without ever bringing our bare feet in contact with the earth.

We often think that grounding requires elaborate rituals, but I personally think that grounding can be as simple as being in contact with the earth: walking on it with bare feet, touching it with your hands, or sitting or stretching your whole body out on the ground. It's undoubtedly an excellent start. Others may prefer more ritual in the form of a meditation or visualisation in addition to make contact with the earth imaginatively as well as physically. Some find that even on a packed subway train or airplane, when direct contact with the earth is impossible, meditation and visualisation can be a comfort.

So, your goal for this month: as often as you can, even if just for five minutes, slip off your shoes and walk on the grass, sand or dirt. Take a moment in your garden or a local park to sit or lay on the ground. If the weather is wet or especially cold, try instead hold and touch objects from the earth – lay your hand on tree bark, pick up fallen pine cones…

If you would like further guidance, why not try these other ideas for grounding?

Body Awareness

When you can't physically touch the earth, giving your body attention can encourage your energy to settle into balance on its own. This is an excellent simple practice to assist that process. Lay your hands on your heart or tummy and spend some time connecting to your body and breath. Take a sweep of awareness from the top of your head to the tips of your toes. In meditation, this is sometimes known as a 'body scan'. You do not have to 'do' anything physical, just take time to check in with the whole body, and let your mind release any areas of tensions, or 'holding.'

Root Meditation

Imagine your energy travelling down through your legs and into the earth. Roots from your feet sink into the soil to draw energy up from the ground. Feel the earth energy flow up into your body, and then send the energy back down and out through your roots. You are creating an energy cycle in order to seek balance.

Exercise

Exercise can help to release any excess energy. And this is where yoga can come in. Grounding in yoga is every bit as important to the practice of yoga as it is to witchcraft. Simple exercises like walking or running in nature, breathing in the fresh air can also help to bring grounding and ease into your life.

Grounding Elements

Crystals, herbs, spices, essential oils and other personal objects can have a grounding effect. They may act as tools to help us achieve a grounded state or help us focus on the element of earth. For example, carnelian crystal, turmeric root and cedarwood oil are all considered beneficial for grounding.

Chakras

You can utilise the chakra system, focusing on the root chakra as part of your grounding exercise. Take a comfortable seat on the grass, earth or rock and visualise connecting the root chakra, at the base of the spine, with the earth.

Grounding for Magic

Grounding before a spell or ceremony can help focus and reduce internal distractions. Grounding after the completion of a ritual or spell helps return us to a calm state. Sometimes a ceremony or spell can leave witches tired, as with any activity that draws our intense focus. We may feel physically and mentally exhausted or a little 'spaced out'. Grounding can help both prevent and remedy this feeling, bringing your mind and energy back into the 'real' world, especially important if you have to walk or drive home!

Grounding before a ceremony is often accomplished through meditation and visualisation. In a group ritual, the leader may lead the participants through a guided meditation to achieve this. Meditations are often combined with 'calling in' of the directions, done as part of the opening (and closing) of many ceremonies. You will learn how to do this in Chapter 12, Ritual and Celebration.

Grounding for Yogis

Feeling grounded is essential, both physically and psychologically, for successful yoga practice (and any mindful practice). In yoga, the word grounding serves as both an adjective (to feel grounded) and a verb, to physically ground down through the feet and hands. To physically ground by bringing awareness into your body helps us find that rooted, stable connection with the earth. So we take time in our practice to notice how feet and hands feel as they make contact with the floor, grounding ourselves fully to build a strong foundation for each asana.

Grounding can also help us achieve calm by directing energy downward, pulling our physical awareness into the 'here and now'. Many of us know the feeling of being all 'in our heads', overthinking, feeling scattered and overwhelmed by the busyness of the world around us. As an airy Libra, I know this feeling very well. In contrast, to be grounded is to be in the moment with a sense of calm and solidity, to balance out the busy moving world with the solid earth. In re-establishing a bond to the earth, we can feel more supported and reminded of our own strength to support ourselves.

Yoga Poses for Groundedness

Tree Pose

Poses of balance like the Tree encourage focus and breath control to find stability. From standing, feet grounded firm into the earth, bring your weight onto your left foot. Next, soften your right knee and open from the hip like a door swinging open. Bring the base of your right foot to the inseam of your left leg and place it on either your inner calf or thigh. Standing tall like a mighty oak, draw your hands to your heart centre and press your palms together. Breathe. It can help to find a still point in the distance to focus on – in yoga we call this the *drishti* point.

Mountain Pose

Stand tall like a mountain. Feet rooted in the earth, rise tall through your body, open your heart and shoulders, and shine the inner creases of your elbows forward. That's it! From the outside, you are a gorgeous mountain, from the inside, you are grounded, powerful and immovable – a force of nature not to be underestimated!

Child's Pose

Dropping your head beneath your heart signals to the nervous system that it's time to slow down and rest, this is why Child's Pose is a very restorative posture. From kneeling, spread your knees out a little wider than your hips and bring your big toes together to touch. Set your bum back to rest on your heels, and walk your palms forward. Rest your forehead on the floor.

Forward Fold

Paschimottanasana, as it is known in Sanskrit, means 'the West', as in the place of the setting sun, so I often think of this pose as one of setting and settling, winding down, and calming the mind. From a seated position, legs extended straight out in front of you, hinge from your hips keeping the spine long. Bring the hands to the legs, lengthen through the torso and let the neck be soft.

Savasana

Corpse Pose is one that promotes deep relaxation. Lie on your back and take a few moments to find comfort in your body. Allow Mother Earth to support you, as you remind yourself that it is safe to let go.

To see these poses and learn more, head to **sentiayoga.com/yoga-forwitches**

Grounding Goddesses

Banbha (Celtic) is the generous Earth Mother, like other well-known earth goddesses Gaia, Pachamama and Terra. She is also the goddess of shelter and stone circles. Connect to Banbha for a blessing of security and grounding, find a stone circle (or any stones that are special to you) in your area. Walk the circle in her honour, connecting to the space in quiet reflection and gratitude, you can request a blessing from the goddess here as well, and leave an offering if you like. For the most eco-conscious items I suggest collecting something on your walk to your stone site, such as a pine cone, berries or fallen leaves and use these as offerings.

Closing Thoughts

For me, in my yoga meditations, I often talk about letting everything beyond our bodies fall away out of our awareness, so that all we are left with are the 'roots' of who we are: body, mind, heart and breath. If I could say just one thing about the specialness of connecting to the earth, it would be to remember that the earth will support you. You already have everything you need: ground beneath your feet, air in your lungs, blood pumping around your body, and fire of heart and mind alive. And although having these things doesn't mean you won't come across struggle, grief, anger and pain, it's always useful to remember that we are strong enough to deal with whatever comes our way. As long as the earth endures, so shall we.

MEDITATION MAGIC

In the story of yoga, meditation came before the balances and handstands. Going back to Patanjali's *Yoga Sutras*, the union that is yoga can only happen when the mind becomes quiet – which is essentially what meditation is. Mental stillness is found by bringing the body, mind and senses to calm, which, in turn, relaxes the nervous system. In an observation as relevant today as it was then, Patanjali suggests that meditation begins when we discover that our never-ending quest to possess things that we believe will meet our craving for pleasure and security can never be completely satisfied. Fulfilment from external sources can never last, so we must turn inwards.

Meditation in Patanjali's eight-limbed system is defined as a state of pure consciousness. The last three limbs of his eight-fold path – *dharana* (concentration), *dhyana* (meditation), and *samadhi* (bliss) – are so closely linked they are collectively referred to as *samyama* (holding together, binding) this is the inner, mental practice of the yogic path. Meditation is used to focus the mind and enter a state of consciousness different from our daily awareness. Meditation can be used to contemplate something affecting us inwardly or outwardly. During this altered state of consciousness, you may feel you can contact your inner self or communicate with the Divine/Universe/Spirit.

Meditation is more commonly associated with yoga and Eastern religions, but it is a core part of magical practice too. It is the starting point for magical techniques such as astral projection and 'hedge riding'.

Meditation is very simple, but not necessarily easy. It can be challenging to quiet the mind, especially within the constant chatter and distractions of a busy world. Some people can meditate for hours, while some feel happy with ten minutes each day. While the aim is not to fall asleep, if you do, know that it is because your body needed the rest. You can combine visualisation and meditation, called guided meditation, visualisation or sometimes journeying, where you picture a scene in your mind's eye. From here, you may imagine something you want, such as seeing yourself relaxed and happy if you feel stressed, or visualising an outcome you are seeking from a project.

Hedge Riding –
The Magic of The Hedge Witch

Here's the thing about the name Hedge Witch, it's probably not the 'hedge' you are thinking of! Not a green planted hedge of a garden that is. Although Hedge Witches do love to be in gardens and forests. Hedge Witch refers to the metaphorical hedge that divides our world with the spirit realm or otherworld. These witches move between the two realms; they use meditation to 'cross over' into other realms, what is sometimes called 'Hedge Riding'. And this is why the Hedge Witch is featuring in this chapter about meditation. Heard of flying witches? It's a prevalent stereotype! One theory of the origin of this idea of witches flying is the Hedge Witch entering altered states of consciousness, often using meditation and thus 'flying' to other worlds: for healing, knowledge, insight, to connect to ancestors, and inspiration for spell work. A Hedge Witch, like a shaman, acts as a mediator between the human world and the spirit world.

The Real Magic of Meditation

In a very real way, you are changing your brain for the better when you meditate. Neuroimaging techniques have shown us that many areas of the brain are affected during and after meditation. With practice, people become calmer, have a higher capacity for empathy and tend to respond to life events in a more balanced way. However, you do have to keep meditating. Why? Just as playing the piano over time stimulates and sustains neural networks involved with playing music. Meditation over time can make us more efficient governors of our own minds, pausing to respond to our worlds instead of mindlessly reacting.

Continued meditation practice ensures that the new neural pathways stay strong. Focused attention is very much like a muscle, one that needs to be strengthened through exercise. Electrical signals in the brain form pathways, these links become stronger the more you repeat a particular behaviour. We know this as a habit. Reaching for a bucket of ice cream each time you have a bad day at work can become a habit. Just as meditation can be.

If you meditate regularly, many positive things happen. These are just a few...

(**Improved focus.** Meditation is a practice in focusing our attention and being conscious of when it wanders. This becomes a lasting effect of regular meditation, even when we are not meditating.

(**The ability to 'tune out' distraction,** which in turn makes for better recall/memory.

(The more we meditate, the **less anxiety** we tend to experience. Brain scan studies have found that the amygdala, the home of our fearful and anxious emotions, decreases in volume after sustained meditation and mindfulness practices. This is because we're loosening the connections of particular neural pathways. This effect can be furthered with positive imagery meditation.

(**More compassion.** As we activate our insula we are more able to experience empathy for others (and at the same time we are calming our amygdala. Making us less likely to react from a place of fear or anger, invaluable in making empathetic choices). Meditating activates the ability to put ourselves in another person's shoes, increasing our ability to feel empathy and compassion for everyone.

(When you encounter a sensation such as stress, fear, anxiety or something potentially upsetting, you can look at it from a **calmer observer perspective** (rather than automatically reacting).

(Improved focus and lower stress allow us to **perform better under pressure** while feeling less stressed.

☾ Meditation **increases brain function** by synchronising the right and left hemispheres of the brain, known as "whole brain synchronisation."

☾ The stimulation that meditation provides the brain **increases dopamine and serotonin levels** – our happiness chemicals.

Simple Ways to Meditate

Whilst the science is helpful to know, you don't need to understand it all to benefit from meditation. These practices are super simple and a great place to start.

Breathing – Focus on the Breath

Meditation is a practice of focus. To meditate on the breath, we focus upon it. So, from a comfortable seat, notice the way the breath feels coming in and out of your nostrils. Notice how it lifts your chest and fills your belly as you inhale. Notice how the belly and chest fall as you exhale. Notice it without judgement. Allow yourself to be with your breath – no need to control it or modify it – just notice it.

I breathe in. I breathe out.

Do this for five minutes – you can set a timer if you like.

Body Scan

Tension within the body and mind are distractions, so we aim to release all tension when meditating. Visualise your whole body as you relax (you can be seated or lying down). With slow, easeful breaths imagine with each exhale of breath you are releasing part of the body into the ground, letting go of tension and tightness. Start with the toes, release and relax them, then the legs and move up the body until you get to the top of your head.

Mindfulness

Mindfulness is a state of awareness in the present moment while greeting and accepting feelings, thoughts, and bodily sensations as they arise. Minds wander, and we can lose touch with our body, engrossed in thoughts, worries and regrets. And that makes us anxious. Mindfulness is the cultivation of the ability to be fully present: to bring our attention back to where we are, bringing the mind to fully attend to what's happening.

Yoga Nidra

Yoga nidra or yogic sleep (*nidra* means 'sleep' in Sanskrit) is a meditation technique. It is all done while resting comfortably lying down in *savasana* (Corpse Pose).

I love nidra because almost anyone can do it. Energetic yoga classes are wonderful but not suitable for everybody: yoga nidra is a practice that everyone can explore. All that you need do is lie down on the floor (or be able to relax in a seated position) and follow the guiding voice of your teacher. It is always guided, so it can be easier for many to focus, helping those whose minds are prone to wandering in meditation practice. Likely you won't remember everything your teacher says as you drift into yogic sleep. It's also very possible you will actually fall asleep! That's okay too. Your unconscious mind is probably absorbing the practice. Or at the very least the body is getting the rest it needs!

Yoga nidra promotes deep rest and relaxation. The stages of relaxation and breath awareness alone can be practised to calm the nervous system, leading to less stress and better health.

This practice can instil a deep sense of peace and relaxation; a space to explore your needs, as well as an opportunity to work on releasing long-held tensions.

The outline of a yoga nidra class can vary, but the main features include a period of relaxation and release of the body, followed by a guided meditation to allow the mind to slip into conscious rest. A yoga nidra practice can be a few minutes or an hour long. I always lead a body scan and then a guided visualisation, to relax the limbs and nervous system, creating a soothing state.

Yoga nidra can also be a spiritual practice of self-study (*svadhyaya*) and a form of *pratyahara* (withdrawal from the senses). When we journey to the deepest workings of our minds in a relaxed and restful state, we may discover insights or inspiration.

You may enjoy making yoga nidra practice part of your regular evening routine, or as a break from a busy day. Witches may use nidra to celebrate an esbat, any ritual, or explore a journey within the mind's eye.

Manifestation and Visualisation

Visualisation and manifestation are practices that have been used in many walks of life to focus and harness the power of the mind and call into being the practitioner's intentions. Studies have shown that when sports people visualise winning a sport or practising a technique in their mind, their performance can improve in real life. You can envision succeeding in a job interview – answering the questions confidently and projecting your true self, and maybe you also visualise yourself working in this new job already. You may wish to cast a spell of 'manifestation' or use visualisation to aid in manifesting practices. Positive visualisation is a 'dress rehearsal' for the brain, creating positive connections with the thought of an event. Neither manifestation nor positive visualisation are guarantees of success, but they can help in many ways, including helping us have a positive mindset and self-belief, and removing conscious and unconscious self-sabotage.

Creating our dreams and desires starts from within. Manifestation as a spell or ritual is about consciously identifying who you want to be and where you want your path to lead. It's about recognising that your thoughts influence your feelings, which in turn can impact your actions, and what you create in your life. The foundation of manifestation is that your beliefs hold immense power and affect how you see the universe.

When manifesting it's often best to focus on the path you seek, rather than specifics. This is especially when it comes to love: you cannot force a particular person to become drawn to you, but you can invite love into your life. Look instead toward finding, for example a relationship that makes you feel safe and loved. Of course, you can get specific if you are really after a particular job, project, house... but be prepared for it not to come to you in the exact form you seek. You may not get *that* job, but have faith that your path will be taking you somewhere better.

Keep it Positive!

When manifesting it should be for good, never try and manifest something terrible to befall someone. Here we fall into the realm of hexes and curses. Whether you think of karma, the Wiccan Rede or prepare for the negative energy to return to you in multiple, I would propose that creating more negativity in this world and in your practice is not wise or useful. By all means get angry if you need, release a tirade of glorious fury by shouting, screaming, throwing things around the room...and then let it go. Holding onto anger can make you bitter, cruel and vengeful. Use a spell to let go of anger and to cut ties with people that have hurt you. But my belief is that you have the power to decide who you are each day, and sending out negative or angry energy in spells is not a healing path to walk down.

Positive Visualisation

Positive visualisation is like a rehearsal for achievement. Visualisation creates and reinforces neural pathways, which prepares our bodies to act consistently with what we visualise. In Sanskrit, you might reference *samskara*, which mean the imprints of our thoughts – they leave a mark in our minds, so use your thoughts wisely! When you mentally rehearse "outcome visualisation" using all your senses to visualise a goal or a "process visualisation" mentally rehearsing the steps you will take, you are putting your mind through a test run.

How to:

Get yourself into a comfortable, relaxing position, readying yourself for meditation.

1. Focus on Your Goal

Decide what you want to focus on for this exercise: it might be a better job, healing from past hurt, more happiness or health.

2. Create a Detailed Picture of That Goal

Visualise your desired outcome as if it is already achieved – and visualise it as happening right now. Visualise yourself in your chosen situation – notice all your senses to build this environment in your mind's eye. See yourself as confident, joyful and authentic.

What do you see? What can you smell/touch/taste? How do you feel in this situation? What qualities are you letting shine – your intelligence, strength, humour? See yourself in this situation, being completely who you wish to be. Include as many details as you can. Fully inhabit your visualised state.

3. Repeat

Repetition adds energy to your visualisation. Try to visualise for a few moments every day. Working towards integrating your visualisation into your current reality.

Manifestation Ritual

I love using candles, so this is a simple candle magic manifestation ritual: the candle can illuminate your intentions and release it outward into the world. You may wish to use a candle that relates to your intention, i.e. yellow for confidence, creativity, optimism, personal power; orange for prosperity, joy and courage; pink for all things love – compassion, friendship, harmony, healing, and self-love; red is for fertility, passion and strength.

(Take time to ground and prepare before you start the ritual.

(Waxing moon to full moon are good times to work manifesting spells.

(You may want to cast a circle (outlined in Chapter 12) or call in the directions/elements.

(You can smudge the space (I like rosemary smudge sticks best, and I make them myself. But you can also use sage).

(Sit comfortably in front of your unlit candle on a heatproof surface like a dish or coaster (possibly at your altar). Have a piece of paper and a pen ready.

(Close your eyes and take deep easeful breaths, focus your attention on your third-eye chakra between your eyebrows.

(Visualise your goals and what you'd like to manifest, actively seeing yourself experiencing this reality and focusing on the sensation of the experience.

(Once you've captured that feeling and have visualised your wish, take out your pen and paper and write down your intention/manifestation; it can be words, drawings, a sigil, a brainstorm – whatever feels right in the moment.

☾ When you are ready, voice your intention, say it out loud into the universe as many times as you like. Then, fold your paper three times and place it underneath the candle dish. Then place your candle on top.

☾ Send the energy of your intention to the candle.

☾ Light the candle, focus on the flame and send your intention into the light. If you wish to say something out loud, you could say, "I light this flame, I ignite this fire. I am ready to manifest all I desire."

☾ When you are ready, extinguish your candle. You can relight it whenever you want to revisit or reinvigorate your intentions, or while you continue to work on bringing your dreams to life. You may replace the candle if it burns out while you are still working on your manifestation.

☾ If you want to create a new intention, or are ready to release an old one, you can light your candle and burn (safely!) the old intention. You may wish to say something like, "With gratitude, I release this intention."

Sigils

A sigil is a picture that represents a desire or intention. They are most commonly created by writing out the intention, then condensing the letters down to form an icon. They are a lovely creative way to illustrate your goals, and a very portable magic – you can draw them in books, on your hands, clothes, into candles, anywhere! In Hindu and yogic culture, images with magical properties are known as yantra, *some yogis meditate on* yantra *to calm and focus their minds.*

Other ways to aid manifestation – practical and magical!

☾ Set out clear goals and take baby steps towards your life goals.

☾ Create a vision board of what you wish to manifest or the life you seek.

☾ Create a witch bottle (shared in Chapter 12) put paper inside the container with the key words you have written down for what you wish to manifest, add a small piece of clear quartz or citrine to the bottle to help boost success and manifest your dreams. Keep the container safe and hidden.

☾ Repeat an affirmation to help keep you focused on your goal and motivation. For example, "I am strong and knowledgeable enough to speak up during meetings." "I enjoy taking steps towards my goals."

Goddesses of the Otherworld

Should you wish to connect to the otherworld and your ancestors to assist you in your meditation or visualisation, wise crone Hecate is a wonderful goddess to work with.

Hecate (Greek) Goddess of crossroads, moon, magic and the underworld. Hecate is the goddess of witchcraft, the original boundary-crosser and hedge rider. Hecate stands at the gateways between realms – earth, heavens and underworld – as both guardian and guide.

Hecate can meet you at the crossroads – be it between choices, paths or worlds. As a crone goddess, she is wise; she has journeyed many lifetimes. She can remind us that there are no wrong or right choices, alleviating the fear that can cause us great indecision. There is no right or wrong, only choice. And by connecting to whatever magic we choose – our inner voice, the wisdom of our ancestors, goddesses, the elements – we can make our choice and step forward along our path with acceptance, and nurture wholeness. There will be challenges, hardships and mistakes along your way, but from it all, you will learn and grow.

Closing Thoughts

Meditation is, all at once, the simplest thing and the hardest thing. It is a letting go and surrendering, but also a connecting and a union to something else – magic? Goddess? The otherworld? Universal consciousness? Spirit? It can be different for everyone, and different every time you meditate. The mind is habitual, old habits can endure if something deeper remains to be discovered. If we are to allow spirituality to unfurl, there needs to be conscious awareness brought to everything we do and think. A meditation practice, then, is not only significant to life, but spiritual and emotional healing journeys too.

As we peel away those layers, like Goddess Inanna losing her layers of clothing as she descended into the underworld, we come to our true selves, letting those layers of fear, anxiety, stress, consumerism and pressure fall away. Perhaps from this place of freedom, we may travel to other realms or visualise our own success. Your body, breath and mind are your finest tools, all that is needed is practice.

MAGIC ON THE MAT

I started this book around the phrase "Find Your Magic on the Mat". Within yoga practice, there are possibilities for daily magic as well as lifelong change. Yoga can lift you up: body, mind, and spirit. As well as providing the roots that can ground you into stability and strength, no matter what comes your way. Your body is the home of the divine essence that is you. Regular yoga practice creates new neural pathways of thinking about your body, mind, heart and spirit. These pathways create inner calm, peace, and presence in the here and now. And that's pretty magical! I've put together some ideas to help you create this magical yoga work, just as you would create a magic spell...

Pranayama

Prana is the life-force that flows through and connects all living things, what others may call *chi*, Goddess, Spirit or Energy of the Universe. We can activate and energise prana through yoga.

When you practice yoga, you are opening up the body to allow this healing prana energy to move around your body.

Pranayama is the yogic practice of controlling of the breath, and in turn, our prana. Yogis have known for centuries – and now medical science is also beginning to discover – that the breath has incredible restorative powers. By controlling the breath in pranayama, ancient yogis found they could alter their state of mind. The pranayama practice I'll describe here creates these effects by slowing the breath. This engages the parasympathetic nervous system, which in turn calms and soothes us. Just watching your breath for several minutes can have a positive influence on your energy levels and mood. You can multiply this effect by using pranayama – breathing exercises tailored to have an impact on specific feelings and conditions.

Traditionally, pranayama is done while sitting on the ground, with the spine straight. But you can sit in a chair or try lying on your back on the floor if that's easier.

Dirga Pranayama – Three-Part Breath

Dirga pranayama or three-part breath is a calming, grounding breathing exercise that helps focus your attention on the present moment. I often teach this simple pranayama at the beginning of yoga classes as a way to transition students from the busyness and noise of their workday into the time they have set aside for their yoga.

☾ Bring your attention to the inhales and the exhales through your nose.

☾ On each inhale, fill the belly up and allow the abdomen to expand with your breath.

☾ Exhale, releasing all the air out from the belly through your nose.

☾ Repeat this deep belly breathing for a few breaths.

☾ Next, inhale, filling the belly up with air, and then draw in a little more breath, causing the ribs to expand.

☾ Exhale, and let the air go first from the rib cage and then from the belly.

☾ Inhale, filling the belly and rib cage up with air. Then bring in just a little more air and let it fill the upper chest, up to the collarbone, causing the heart centre to rise and expand.

☾ Exhale, and let the breath go first from the upper chest, allowing the heart centre to fall, then from the rib cage, then from the belly.

☾ This is our three-part breath.

☾ Continue at your own pace, as you practice it will feel more easeful.

Bhramari Pranayama – Humming Bee Breath

In *bhramari pranayama*, we create humming, buzzing sounds during exhalation, thought to calm nerves and tension – this is sound healing without the Sanskrit!

(Keep the mouth closed and teeth apart.

(Plug both the ears with your thumbs. You can either use your fingers to rest over the eyes or on top of the head.

(Take a slow deep breath to fill the lungs.

(Exhale slowly, through the nose, making a continuous humming sound from the throat.

(Feel the sound vibration within your head.

(This is one round.

(Try five rounds and see how you get on!

Mudras

If prana is magic moving around our bodies, then mudras are the spells! A mudra is a symbolic gesture performed with the hands and fingers. It creates a 'seal' that facilitates a flow of energy in the body that helps generate a state of mind. Mudras are used in Ayurveda, yoga and meditation for healing, energy and focus. Mudras, used alongside pranayama exercises can invigorate the flow of prana in the body and our hands are all the tools we need.

Just as in spell work, intention is everything. The symbolism of the mudra is most important. My favourite mudra when I am in meditation is the *dhyana mudra*, a gesture that promotes the energy of meditation, contemplation and unity with higher energy. It is formed with upturned hands overlapping one another with the thumbs lightly touching. Anyone who has been to a yoga class may well recognise the *anjali mudra*, or 'prayer hands'. It is often done at the end of the class when we say together "Namaste". It is a hand gesture used to greet another being with respect and acknowledgement for the Divine in us all.

In the book, *Hatha Yoga Pradipika*, mudras are described as having the power to awakening the sleeping serpent goddess of kundalini energy. So I strongly encourage the exploration mudras when connecting to the goddess! A simple mudra that invokes the goddess of fearlessness, inner strength, and empowerment: Kali, is the *Kali mudra*. Bring your hands together interlacing fingers, extend your index fingers. This creates a shape is intended to represent the sword of mighty warrior Kali. But if it also reminds you of Charlie's Angels, then that's all good with me!

The *prana mudra* stimulates the root chakra, empowering and awakening the body, with a boost of prana energy. Each finger on the hand represents an element, and this mudra brings together water, earth and fire elements. Touch the tips of your ring finger and little finger to your thumb. Leave your index and middle finger extended. Keep your eyes closed and focus on your breath. You can do prana mudra while sitting down in a meditative position or while standing in Tadasana. This mudra benefits everything from fatigue and nervousness in the body to enhance self-confidence and improving circulation.

Yoga Asana

Just as you may use spell work or ritual to help soothe a broken heart, to release anger or to aid sleep, yoga asana have their own 'recipes', strings of poses to help energise, heal and/or soothe. You may want to add these moves to your ritual or use them to prepare for one. I will just list the poses here, and should you wish to see them in more detail, you can head to **sentiayoga.com/yogaforwitches**

Yoga for a Broken or Heavy Heart

These four yoga asana can help aid in soothing your heart or help to lift your spirits and find a little peace. Tend to, open, and heal your heart space.

- ☾ **Child's Pose** – rest in this safe space, connect to your breath and the beat of your heart.

- ☾ **Sphinx** – open your heart and let your gaze rise gently.

- ☾ **Reclining Goddess** – which you can do over a bolster or pillow.

- ☾ **Easy Seat** – sit with it, no need to push or challenge, just breathe.

Yoga for Sleep

Move slowly and peacefully as your body and mind recognise this practice as a transition time: a threshold into rest and to sleep.

- ☾ **Forward Fold** – allow the spine to be long as you melt forward and down.

- ☾ **Waterfall** or legs up the wall – you can wiggle your feet and toes if that feels soothing.

- ☾ **Twisted Roots/Supine Twist** – allow gravity to help you wring out through your centre.

- ☾ **Savasana** – settle into the earth.

Yoga to Release Anger

If you're feeling worked up, it might be useful to avoid deep stretching poses, as it's possible you could throw yourself too strongly into poses and pull something. Instead, we'll look at releasing energy, grounding and drawing focus to breath and balance.

☾ **Lion's Roar** from seated – as you exhale, roar out your rage! Stick out your tongue and look to the skies!

☾ **Arm Sweeps** – raise arms on the inhale and release on the exhale.

☾ **Mountain Pose** – stand rooted into the earth, stand tall and strong like a mountain.

☾ **Tree Pose** – finding a focus as you continue to root into the earth.

If you are still feeling an excess of energy, you may want to roll through a few rounds of Sun Salutations as well.

Namaste, Witches

How about bringing a little witchcraft into your yoga practice? Here are some ideas:

☾ *Let a candle burn during your yoga practice. Anoint a purple candle with clary sage and jasmine oil to connect to inner wisdom and the third eye chakra.*

☾ *'Call in the Directions' during your opening meditation or practice a Sun Salutation in each of the four directions, turning a full circle with four rounds.*

☾ *Smudge your yoga practice space with sage or rosemary.*

☾ *Place crystals around your mat. For example, rose quartz for peace and tranquility during your practice. Or one of my favourites, citrine, which helps to improve concentration and focus, clearing your mind for your practice.*

Goddesses of Mantra and Meditation

Sarasvati (Hindu) Goddess of music, learning and writing, she is considered the inventor of the Sanskrit language. 'Sarasvati' refers to both a goddess and an ancient sacred river in India's mythology. As the personification of this sacred river and water in general, Sarasvati represents everything that flows: music, poetry, writing, learning and dance.

Green Tara (Buddhist) Tara is a Bodhisattva – a compassionate, enlightened being. She has twenty-one forms, each one with a different colour and spiritual attribute. Of these twenty-one forms, two are particularly popular – White Tara, associated with compassion and long life, and Green Tara, associated with enlightened activity and abundance. Tara has her own mantra, often used in her honour:

om tare tuttare ture soha

"I bow to the liberator and protectress"

Green Tara's hands are often portrayed in symbolic mudras such as the *varada mudra*, the gesture of giving. Made with the hand extended and facing downward, with the palm facing out, it expresses the energy of compassion and acceptance.

Closing Thoughts

"Can we make time for ourselves where there is nothing we have to do? No roles we have to play? And just be..."

At about this point, when I say these words in my meditation class, someone will be checking their smartwatch or examining their fingernails. And I send them a little love. To 'just be' is a simple concept, but that does not make it easy. So...we practice. It's all we can do.

Maybe we try yoga nidra, mantra or pranayama to help bring our mind to quiet, and let those distractions of the world fall away a little. Can you allow everything outside of the microcosm on your mat that is your body, sink into soft focus? Can you allow yourself to 'switch off'? It's not easy, but meditation, nidra, mantra and mudra can all help us find this peace, nothing more or less than the next inhale and exhale... It is from this place that we may wish to manifest, cast spells, rest, or experience the moment.

Yoga (and indeed witchcraft) invite us to peel away the layers of life and discover: Who are we when we are not afraid? When we are not stressed? When we are not distracted by concerns of emails, schedules, timetables...? Of course, these layers build up, and that's okay, this is part of being human. But take some time as often as you can to peel away, step out of your layers and reconnect to your essence, energy, magic: your body, breath and heart.

MAGIC WORDS

The use of magic words – both those we write down and those we speak aloud – lie at the heart of magical practice and also many yoga practices. What we say and how we say it holds great power: the energy of our words is one of our greatest magics. In this chapter we'll first explore the ancient power of the language of yoga: Sanskrit. Before moving into the magical uses of writing and speaking.

Sanskrit

In India, Sanskrit is considered divine – spoken by gods and capable of connecting us mere mortals with the transcendent self. The word Sanskrit means "completely formed; hallowed; refined". Each word is considered a *bija*, or seed mantra. The essential meaning of each word and letter in the Sanskrit alphabet is thought to be contained within its sound. The sounds of the Sanskrit language are believed to have a healing effect, as well as leading to transformation and channelling of spiritual light.

I think many sounds can be healing, balancing the mind and the body. A Sanskrit scholar from England – Sir John Wodrof (aka Arthur Avalon) lived in India at the time of British rule, and he describes ancient texts depicting the presence of the sounds of the Sanskrit language actually present in the centres of the energy body (the chakras).

In guiding students through yoga classes and meditation, the words I use bind the class together. I provide guidance for the poses and breathwork, the opportunity to reflect, as well as encouragement and advice. It's a lot to weave together: to hold space with words. But I find that as long as I speak from the heart, it all works out okay!

Mantra

Ayurvedic medicine considers mantra repetition to be one of its best tools for bringing about greater health. A combination of the healing language of Sanskrit and the ability of mantras to help focus the mind means the process of chanting can restore body, mind and health to wholeness. There are mantras for connecting to each of the major chakras of the body.

Simple mantras can be added to meditation, ritual or breathwork. In Sanskrit, *man* is 'mind', and *tra* is 'free from'. Mantras can be used as a tool to free the mind, allowing the conscious mind to relax. The use of dedicated mantra for some time not only switches up your practice and gives you something to focus on, but can also help you get out of the internal dialogue of the mind. It's about bringing intention and awareness to the sound.

I won't try and teach you any elaborate chants here, it's not something I am an expert on (but there are many learned teachers out there if you do wish to learn more). But I want to share a few ideas to get you thinking.

One of the best-known bija mantras is *Om*, the vibration and primordial sound.

Om was the first sound of the universe in Hindu mythology, so it represents the birth, death and re-birth process. You may feel or envisage the energy of the sound lifting from your root up through to the top of your head at the crown chakra. The sound of *Om* can unblock the throat chakra and encourage more attuned communication with others.

As we saw in Chapter 2, there is a specific seed sound for each of the chakras.

One slightly longer mantra that you might chose to use in Sanskrit or English is:

lokah samastah sukhino bhavantu

"May all beings be happy and free,
and may the thoughts, words, and actions of my own life
contribute in some way to happiness and freedom for all."

Simple Mantras

Mantras don't need to be long, formal or complicated. You can choose any mantra (in any language you wish) such as: "Breathe", "Relax" or "It is safe to let go".

Mantras

☽ I can and I will.

☽ Everything I need is within me.

☽ I am love.

☽ I am strong.

☽ I am beautiful/I am working towards finding my beauty.

☽ I give myself permission to…

☽ My potential is unlimited.

☽ I release what no longer serves me.

Sankalpa

A *sankalpa* is an intention or declaration of desire, e.g. "Today I will forgive" or "Today I will be kind". You may be asked at the beginning of a yoga class to set a *sankalpa*, and keep it in mind during your practice. It is a personal vow from you to the universe. We plant seeds of intention at the beginning of the practice and nourish and nurture them so they can take root and grow.

You may also choose to say your *sankalpa* out loud or internally in the morning when you rise and at night before you go to bed. Or anytime through the day to help you live with intention.

Writing

Writing is a beautiful way to create simple and amazing magic – taking our thoughts from mind to page. It doesn't have to be great poetry or prose; it doesn't have to be for anyone but yourself. There's magic in writing: it can be cleansing, enriching, and grounding. It allows us to process the emotions and experiences of our life, creating reminders of times when you have achieved great things, learned new things and encountered wonder. We are creating, in writing, visual representations of what we've survived and thrived through.

The ways to implement writing into your life are endless: writing as a form of manifesting, reflections or reminders.

The practice of journal writing dates back to the days when our ancestors wrote on cave walls, making sense of our world by recording it. A journal can play many roles: a tool for self-expression, clarity, creativity, and an exploration of what you think and feel. For something so simple, there are a fantastic number of benefits linked to journaling from calming anxiety and stress to increasing mental clarity, creativity, awareness and spiritual growth.

Journaling is a tool that yogis may call *svadhyaya* or self-study. Your journal, like your mat, can be a sanctuary, and place of reflection. As you look over what you are writing take time to reflect: are you holding onto anger or frustrations? Are you blaming others? Are you missing solutions that are available to you?

Meditation and Journaling: Combining Practices

By exploring our inner world through meditation and journaling, we can utilise both practices for deeper reflection and connection. Both meditation and journaling create a space for exploration: we are not trying to change or criticise, but just to observe and note thoughts, and feelings as they arise. Something that we have real difficulty with in modern life is stopping, reflecting or meditating: taking time to do nothing. It is easy to forget the value of doing nothing. Finding that space and silence is essential. It's only in quieting body and mind (*chitta vritti nirodha*) that we allow space for inspiration, growth and relaxation. Allow yourself to pause from the busyness of life to explore, discover and learn from your inner world.

When we put thoughts to paper in our journal, we can clear our mind and gain perspective. By combining meditation and journaling, you can access deeper wisdom and cultivate a greater understanding of your experiences and what you can learn from them.

Journal Prompts

You may wish to write whatever comes to mind or spend a few minutes of free writing. Sometimes questions, mantras or quotes can help get you started. Here are a few ideas:

Questions

☾ How can I nourish my inner goddess today?

☾ Am I moving in a direction I want to go in?

☾ How are my choices helping my happiness?

☾ How can I better support my goals?

☾ How can I practice self-care today?

☾ What magic is present in my morning?

☾ What am I grateful for?

☾ Do I have an intention for this day?

☾ What seasonal abundance is present in nature today?

☾ What do I feel drawn to achieve?

☾ Is anything holding me back?

☾ What does my dream day look like?

Writing Spells

A spell is a focused intention and harnessed energy – we might also know these as prayers or manifestations. A spell can consist of a set of words, a verse, a ritual action, or any combination of these. Spellcasting can be as simple or complex as you want it to be. You can use as many ingredients and tools as you'd like. Seek guidance from books, the internet and friends, and experiment for yourself. Note down what works for you and what doesn't.

More than anything a spell is about focusing your attention on where you want to direct your energy. A spell can undoubtedly help you on the journey towards a goal, but you will also have to work towards that goal. You can create a spell for anything you wish. The words may feel divinely inspired or just what comes to mind (often that is one and the same).

Your words hold meaning, so think about what it is you want: to let go, self-love, to forgive… Then using other elements of ritual such as opening and closing a circle or meditation, you have the building blocks to create a spell and ritual all of your own! But remember, the words, the herbs and candles, the tools – these are all to focus your own energy. The most essential witchcraft tool is your mind.

Here is a simple outline of a spell and ritual

☾ Reflect on your journal notes. What would you like to connect to in order to thrive? Let's say you identify self-love and self-acceptance as an area in your life you want to nurture.

☾ On a full moon night prepare a simple potion of Love Goddess tea. (Recipe in Chapter 7).

☾ Open your Circle or Call in a Circle (see Chapter 12).

☾ Draw down the moon (see Chapter 9).

☾ Say a simple spell you have prepared. (This is one I have written, you can write your own).

"Goddesses of the Moon; Selene, Hina, Artemis,
Help me embrace my body as a source of joy and beauty,
Help me care for myself as I care for others,
Help me embrace my inner goddess.
I am beautiful and deserving of love, I am beautiful and deserving of love, I am beautiful and deserving of love.
Blessed Be!"

☾ Drink your tea.

☾ While you sip your tea, write in your journal ten things that make you feel beautiful, i.e. dancing, singing, laying in the sunshine, massage, getting a manicure, laughing with friends…

☾ Maybe draw an oracle card for any advice from the goddesses as you set out on your path of self-love.

☾ You may wish to commit to taking an action of self-love each day, maybe drawing from your list. Perhaps take a moment at your altar each day to light a candle or reflect on your spell and your path.

☾ Open the Circle.

☾ Continue on your journey…

As with all things, time, patience and love are what is needed to bring your intentions and spells to life!

Book of Shadows

A Book of Shadows — also called a Grimoire — is a place for a witch to keep their spells, rituals and ideas. So, just like a journal...but for witches! It includes anything you would like to note down or keep for inspiration: recipes, potions, herb blends, moon phases, goals — anything worth taking note of. Your Book of Shadows can physical or digital. (Mine is covered in golden hearts and has coloured ribbons dividing the sections). There are no solid rules as to what you can place in your Book of Shadows. If you are part of a coven or grove, your peers may have suggestions. But, as this is your book, and one that needn't be shown to anyone else, it's really up to you.

Cast Away

You can bring writing magic into a yoga class, or any group environment you are part of. This simple ritual is particularly lovely for the new moon, after a focused meditation (which is how I do it). On a piece of paper, write down anything you would like to let go of this month. Then scrunch up your paper and cast it away with intention – for example, burn, bury or smudge it.

When guiding this activity in yoga classes, I ask my students to put the scrunched up pieces of paper into a cauldron or bowl. Then when I get home I smudge and burn the 'letting go' items, as it's not usually practical to do that in a yoga studio! As I tell my yoga students, magic like yoga is all about intention. Here in this super simple ceremony, we acknowledge, with intention, that which we wish to let go of and then intentionally let it go into the cauldron. We move forward with our new intentions. It's precisely the same when you move, balance, and breathe in yoga – you need intention – you can't just throw yourself into a headstand asana and hope for the best. That's how people get hurt! No, we move the body and the breath with intention to-wards our goal of feeling a little calmer, maybe a little more balance at the end of practice. Intention is everything. You have to choose consciously, "I am going to move into this pose, I am going to let go of doubt, I am going to channel this goddess today".

And your mind can wander over time, whether that's over the space of a class or over a month as you forget that you intended to act with more self-love. So you come back, you try again, with intention. You return to your altar, cauldron, mat… That's the circle, the Wheel of the Year, the cycle of our days: there's always a chance to come back and try again.

Freewriting

In freewriting you get out a piece of paper and start to write…and that's it. Just keep writing, pen to paper, without worrying about grammar or punctuation or sentence structure, or even making sense. Creativity requires a free flow of ideas. Through freewriting anyone can jump into this flow and see where it takes us.

In the nineteenth century, freewriting was popular with mediums and spiritualists as a tool to connect with ghosts and other other-worldly beings. But all of us can use it to connect to our conscious and unconscious mind. The 'rule' of freewriting is simply to keep your hand moving, continual movement is key to the success of the practice, before your internal critic or doubts censure ideas.

We often don't have enough of a chance in our culture to do this kind of thing. We're expected to produce, but we're not often given the creative space we need– and this space is vital. It's where we play and experiment, where we make connections and form thoughts. Creativity happens in open, liminal space, and freewriting is great way into that magical space.

Creating your Own Code

You may be aware of the Wiccan Rede and similar witchy codes of "An' ye harm none, do what ye will." Patanjali created the eight limbs as his rule book for yoga. As we explore new avenues of finding magic though yoga, witchcraft and goddesses, you may consider writing your own code, based on the inspiration and ideas you have found here and within yourself. It can be a list of reminders, affirmations or a manifesto of how you wish to live your life moving forward. Whatever form your code or declaration takes, put it somewhere that you can see daily. It might include statements such as:

☾ I am powerful.

☾ I am connecting to my inner strengths every day.

☾ I am as compassionate to myself as I am to others.

☾ I rise by lifting others.

☾ I allow myself to rest when I need it.

☾ I am worthy of every good thing that comes my way.

☾ I will never try to harm someone, be it via magic, spells, social media or by gossiping.

☾ I will try not to judge: everyone is working through their own troubles.

☾ Every day when I wake, I can choose the kind of human/witch/yogi I want to be.

Writing Goddesses

Seshet (Egyptian) Goddess of wisdom, knowledge, and writing, a scribe, record keeper, 'Mistress of the House of Books' and creatrix of writing. In Egyptian lore words possessed a magical power, and many written spells can be found in ancient Egyptian texts. Seshet also became goddess of accounting, architecture, astronomy and astrology. She is often shown holding a palm stem, recording of the passing of time, especially the lifetime of the pharaoh.

Feel free to invent your own writing, like Seshet for your journaling and Book of Shadows. You may want to use symbols, colours, doodles, images from magazines or a combination of all these things to express yourself in your journal pages. Your words, once written down, are protected by Goddess Seshet.

Benzaiten (Japanese) Goddess of everything that flows: water, words, speech, eloquence, music and knowledge. This fluid nature means she is generally associated with the ocean; many of her shrines are located near water, and she is frequently depicted accompanied by a sea dragon. It's suggested that Benzaiten is the Japanese personification of the Hindu goddess Sarasvati, who also represented these flowing elements of music, poetry and writing. Perhaps before you settle at your journal each morning, you take a moment to ask Benzaiten or Sarasvati or set an intention to let your words flow – and just see what comes up.

Closing Thoughts

Celebrate your words, they are your magic. Speak your magic, write down your magic. Your words do not have to be perfect or eloquent or read or heard by anyone but yourself. Write for you, write to make your mark, write for joy and write for sorrow: let your words express the fullness of your magic!

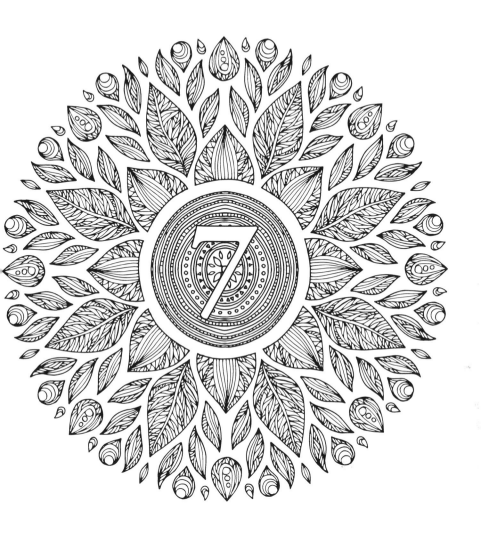

DAILY MAGIC

When you think of magic do you think elaborate costumes and props? Careful pronunciation of spells in old books? Chances are when you think yoga you also think special clothes, albeit of a different kind and expensive props in the form of mats, blocks, bolsters... These notions can keep us from practicing every day, or even put us off all together; as it all seems a little too much work!

I'd like to introduce you to how can we integrate the magic of yoga and witchcraft easefully, into the most commonplace parts of our day – eating, moving and cleaning. We can connect to the nature and energy of magic in little, simple ways throughout our day, making our practice easy and fun!

Who you are can change from day to day. Some days you are warrior goddess, sometimes you feel delicate and vulnerable. Magic and yoga can meet you wherever you are each and every day.

Know that this is a journey and you are making great progress, even if you are not sure who you are today. Ask yourself simple questions – what could nourish me right now? Food, rest, sitting on the grass in the sun, rather than an asana or meditation? Well then that is your first step. Today you are someone that needs to rest, to ground, to sit in the sun. Sometimes it may feel like a confusing world of contradictions: how can I stand in my witchy power and still not know who I am today? How can I send out positive energy and still accept some people will think what I do is devilish/weird/crazy? I know, it's challenging. But we are such complex beings, in an infinitely complex universe.

In yoga class, I often remind my students we can be peaceful and powerful, calm yet strong – all in the same breath. I think there is a peace to be found in the acceptance of all these contradictory powers within us. Finding a way to stand within this unknown and unknowable.

We are gloriously complex and contradictory in a world that loves boxes, snap judgments and 100% certainty. People may find this inability to define you uncomfortable, but this is a reminder that you do not owe anyone an explanation. Your rich inner world needn't mean anything to anyone but yourself. A person can be called a witch for merely knowing, and for owning her knowledge. And to some, for strange reasons that may include fear, power, jealousy, a woman who 'knows' is dangerous indeed. Why? Because she knows different? She knows better? Or is merely aware that no one can know for sure how our world works and she has found her own path and knows it is right for her? Considering the many restrictions placed on women and their bodies in America and other countries of the world right now – maybe it's also about choice. Communicating *I am knowledgeable, powerful, and I can make choices about how I use these strengths*...can be a real challenge to the status quo!

Transformation of consciousness starts with the smallest of steps, simple changes, inviting in of magic. Starting our journey from exactly where we are: in these bodies, in these homes, in this world, at this time of history. Not in our fantasy body in expensive leggings in a perfect house. But here and now. Just start, my dear brave one! Don't think about perfection, or performance, but about creating small sparks that might just lead you into magic and perhaps, great changes.

The Kitchen Witch

The kitchen can be a sacred space where magic is created, whether it's mixing up a potion, or baking a cake with love. The whole process is part of this spell – the intention being just as important as the ingredients! The Kitchen Witch keeps a warm and happy home infused with magic.

Kitchen witchcraft is the magic of hearth and home. This, one of the oldest forms of magic, is growing in popularity as homemakers embrace their inner Kitchen Witch. The Kitchen Witch steeps herbs for remedies or offerings to the spirits, in ancient times she may, while stoking the fire, have sought blessings from the Goddess for a kind winter.

For many, kitchen witchery is getting back to the roots of witchcraft. Back when women and men practised witchcraft at their hearth-fires in ancient dwellings, and to whom people turned to for help and healing. Kitchen Witch, Green Witch, Hedge Witch – are all terms for those witches who do not follow a religion or coven but who prefer to work on their own.

Intention is everything – prepare cheese on toast with love and gratitude, and it too can become a recipe for love, abundance and prosperity!

Bringing a little spark of magic to everyday tasks is a great way to bring more magic to your day. A Kitchen Witch raids her kitchen for her magical tools. Making it easy and cheap to explore, no fancy props needed! A cooking pot is your cauldron, and a wooden spoon is your wand! In her work the lines between the magic and 'real-life' blur as a spark of magic arrives into household chores, which is something I love about the practice.

Two Simple Tea Potions from the Kitchen Witch

Sun Magic Lemon Tea

A simple tea to draw in the power of sunshine, this cleansing and purifying tonic can help with digestion. Lemon water can be a remedy for all manner of colds, fevers, sore throats and general congestion. It's also associated with both the sun and the moon, and so works well with the yoga magic in Chapters 9 and 10.

You will need:

☾ The juice of one fresh, organic lemon.

☾ One lemon slice or sliver of peel to go in the cup.

☾ One teaspoon of honey or maple syrup to sweeten.

Method

1. Serve with boiling water in your favourite cup.

2. Let the warmth of the tea in your hands and at your lips be a moment to pause and enjoy.

Simples

This type of mixture/spell is known as a 'simple': it involves just one ingredient, a magical herb or the mixture made from one. Other fabulous simples include:

☾ *Mint tea for digestion, healing, strength and luck.*

☾ *Chamomile for purification, protection and sleep.*

☾ *Rosemary for power, healing and protection.*

Some, such as mint, lemon and chamomile tend to be taken steeped in water. They may be drunk as a tea or added to a bath or soaking water for feet or hands. Others, such as rosemary or calendula can be added to oil and ingested or massaged into the skin, or infused into alcohol as a tonic. You can make rosemary tea, but I actually prefer a nice rosemary infused gin! You can also add it to olive oil and drizzle over salad and pizzas! (Maybe have the gin and the pizza together, just to be sure!)

Love Goddess Tea

With this drinkable potion we seek the energy of the goddesses of love: Áine, Freya and Aphrodite, inviting love into our lives, in all its forms. Áine was famed for her herbal elixirs of healing. And this one is sweet and gorgeous, featuring correspondences for the goddess Freya: strawberries and mint. In folk magic strawberries symbolise passion and fertility, ideal for a love spell! And mint, named after a seductive Greek nymph, is often used in spells for love, prosperity and healing. This tea potion is sweetened with Aphrodite's favourite ambrosia: honey. Bees and their honey were sacred to the Goddess.

Brew your Love Goddess Tea during the waxing moon, or on Goddess Freya's day – Friday.

You will need:

☾   A sprig of fresh washed mint.

☾   A handful of ripe strawberries, sliced (you can buy dried if needed).

☾   Honey – see if you can find honey from local hives.

☾   Hot water.

Method

1. Simmer strawberries gently for at least ten minutes in a pan with three cups of water.

2. Sieve into your chosen mug.

3. Place the mint sprig into the cup. Drizzle in the honey and stir.

4. Take your time enjoying your tea! As you drink it, envisage drawing love into your day, and life.

Ayurveda

The knowledge of how to utilise herbs and flowers is as old as humanity itself – with formal records dating back 4,000 years. Cultures in ancient Sumeria, India, and China were all known to use herbal remedies.

Ayurveda is a holistic wellness system based on restoring the balance between mind, body and spirit, using dietary and herbal treatments (just like the Green Witch and Kitchen Witch!). Developed in India over thousands of years, Ayurveda is considered one of the world's oldest health modalities and yoga's sister science. Ayurveda, like yoga, is ancient, but its teachings are just as relevant to modern-day life as they have ever been.

Taking its name from combining *ayur* (life) with *veda* (science),

Ayurveda is based on the understanding that we all embody elements of earth, air, fire, water and space. By balancing these elements within us, we can find wellbeing.

The three *doshas* or energetic forces in Ayurveda are known as *Vata, Pitta,* and *Kapha.* They are derived from the five elements, and are forces of nature that exist both within us and in the makeup of the universe. These elements can help us to understand ourselves and the world around us better. And influence our individual physical, mental, and emotional character traits. As well as our unique powers and weaknesses.

Vata encompasses air and ether (think light, flowing, unpredictable).

Pitta is fire and water (powerful, transformational, bold).

Kapha is earth and water (grounded, calm, restorative).

We are all a combination of all three doshas in varying amounts.

We are born with a unique doshic constitution which is called our *prakriti* (which means literally, nature). Our *vikruti* is the doshic constitution we have right now, and it is affected by our environment, stress, diet, sleep patterns, and many other variables.

You may, for example, be born with a *Vata* constitution but be more *Pitta* and fiery during a stressful work project, or you may be more *Kapha* and grounded during winter.

In a yoga class, the fiery *Pittas* are the ones practising lots of handstands, planks and sun salutations. And if someone is feeling particularly *Kapha,* they'll be the first to settle into Savasana and relaxation!

This might be a bit of an exaggeration, but the Ayurvedic *doshas* allow us to see the world, and ourselves, through a whole new lens of elemental energy.

	About	Temperament	In Balance	Unbalanced
Vata **Air +** **Space/** **ether**	Vata embodies the energy of movement and is associated with air and space: clear, creative and flexible. Vata energy is movement: the flow of the breath, the beat of the heart, movement of muscles, tissues and cells. It coordinates communication throughout the mind and nervous system.	Thinly built frame, dry and thin hair and skin. High energy for short periods of time, need plenty of rest.	Inspirational and enthusiastic.	Anxiety and fearfulness.
Pitta **Fire +** **Water**	Pitta represents the fiery energy of transformation and watery energy of movement. Pitta can be unstable, but spreads – much as the warmth of a fire, or as water flows. Pitta is related to intelligence, understanding, digestion of foods, thoughts, emotions, and experiences.	Medium frame, warm complexion, sensitive to sunlight, normal to fine hair. Motivated with focused endurance.	Strong heart, motivated, courageous and driven.	Aggressive, irritable, controlling and judgemental.
Kapha **Earth** **+** **Water**	Kapha brings structure, weight and solidity, associated with the earth and water elements. Kapha embodies the watery energies of love and compassion. This dosha hydrates all cells, lubricating joints and skin, and protecting tissues.	Larger frame, pale complexion, normal to oily hair and skin. Contented temperament with high endurance.	Strong, loving, patient and forgiving.	Irritable, lethargic, greedy and possessive.

We are all different, and finding our own elements and the mix of elements is important. You can learn more about your dosha, with online quizzes such as the one at pukkaherbs.com. They base their tea blends around the principles of Ayurveda.

Daily Routine

The tradition of *dinacharya* (daily routine) is a powerful Ayurvedic tool for improving health and wellbeing. And even if you are brand new to Ayurveda, simple daily actions for health can be easy and pleasant to put in place. For me, warm water and lemon is a lovely way to ease into my day. Here are some other simple daily rituals from Ayurveda.

Meditation, Prayer, or Quiet Reflection

The purpose of a morning routine is to calm the nervous system and ground yourself before the day begins. Meditation, pranayama, prayer, or quiet reflection can help get you there, stilling that *chitta vritti*. You may already have a practice that you enjoy. If not, sitting and breathing slowly and deeply for a few minutes can be a simple and beautiful start.

Yoga

As the 'sister science' of Ayurveda, yoga is a natural part of an Ayurvedic daily routine. Ayurveda would suggest that different individuals will benefit from different types of yoga. Depending on their doshas and current state of balance. If you are *Kapha* seeking a little fire to spark your morning try Sun Salutations. If you are an airy *Vata* seeking grounding try Earth Salutations and grounding seated postures. If you are a fiery *Pitta* in need of soothing, calming meditation and pranayama may be the thing for you.

Because the essence of a daily routine is to support your system in returning to balance, adopting a daily routine is an act of self-love, setting the tone for our entire day. Our routine provides us with an opportunity to prioritise our wellbeing, a reminder that we are worthy of loving attention every day.

One thing that stands out about the ideal Ayurvedic daily routine is its focus on the early morning hours. Many recommended practices are done upon waking, before breakfast. Many of us may know the peace and serenity that is accessible in the hours before sunrise. The early morning hours are a powerful time to engage in loving self-care and reflection. So, an Ayurvedic practitioner may recommend that we rise during the "ambrosial hours" of the morning, before sunrise between 3 am and 6 am (gah!) This is an airy *Vata* time of day: the atmosphere is light and clear, conducive for creating a connection with our deepest inner consciousness. So…I'm a real human, and I would say for many real humans starting your morning routine at 3 am is both distressing and impossible. (I can also share that in my dosha is *Kapha*, the earthy grounded one, so you know, just leave me on the ground at 3 am, I'm fine here thanks!) But what you can take away from this is to rise a little earlier than everyone else in the household. Even if it's just setting your alarm ten minutes earlier, you can take those extra minutes to meditate, draw an oracle card or quietly drink tea and claim the day as your own. Connect to the voice of your spirit before the noise of the day can distract you or drown it out.

Embracing an Ayurvedic lifestyle can be as simple as these easy practices and ideas that can become part of your self-care routine:

☾ Drinking lemon water to start your day and ignite your *agni* (digestive fire).

☾ Make lunch the biggest meal of the day as your digestive fire is at its peak with the sun highest in the sky.

☾ Go for a walk in nature. In Ayurvedic terms, walking is a tri-doshic exercise: it balances all the doshas without putting strain on the body. It can also calm the mind. Go with a friend to catch up on some soul connection too!

☾ Deep breathing or pranayama. Mindful breath improves the flow of oxygen and other vital nutrients to the body.

☾ Go to bed early. Ayurveda emphasises the value of good sleep; rest is the basis of our ability to take dynamic activity. (It's that balance between yin and yang we all need!)

☾ Rise with the sun (optional!) Waking up early gives you time to concentrate and reflect, to prepare a nourishing breakfast. And time to enjoy the early morning calm of nature.

☾ Utilise spice: turmeric, cumin, coriander, fennel, cardamom… Used in Ayurvedic cooking, these, among other spices, add aroma and flavour but also healing goodness to your food.

Yogi Tea

The Ayurvedic respect for the healing properties of vegetables, spices and herbs is very similar to the ideas of the Kitchen Witch. Our food can bring us healing, strength and comfort.

I first had this recipe at a tea and spice plantation in Sri Lanka, a beautiful yoga retreat destination where we moved, swam, explored and sipped much tea! The warming spice blend is based on an Ayurvedic formula of spices to ward off colds and infections. Generations of yogis have drunk this tea to support their meditation and long hours in cold mountain retreats. You can enjoy it anytime you need warming up (I owe many an early morning writing session on dark February mornings to this tea!)

Ginger: Ayurvedic practitioners use ginger for a wide variety of health applications including digestive support and warming the body.

Cardamom: used to support a healthy stomach and digestive function.

Cinnamon: cinnamon bark comes from a small evergreen tree that is native to Sri Lanka. Most other 'cinnamon' we buy in shops is actually cassia bark (so I always get my yogi tea and cinnamon from Sri Lanka). Real cinnamon supports the function of the respiratory, digestive systems and immune function.

Clove: another warming spice, clove buds are the aromatic dried flower buds of a tree in the myrtle family. Clove supports circulation and digestion.

Coriander: coriander seeds can help support and soothe the stomach.

Pepper: black pepper is an important healing spice in Ayurveda. It has cleansing and antioxidant properties, enhancing digestion and circulation. It helps transport the benefits of other herbs to the different parts of the body.

For two mugs you will need:

☾ 7 whole cloves

☾ 10 black peppercorns

☾ 1 or 2 sticks of cinnamon

☾ 10 whole cardamom pods (split pods first)

☾ 4 ginger slices (no need to peel)

☾ 1/4 teaspoon of black tea, or one tea bag

☾ 4 cups of water

☾ Honey or maple syrup to taste

Method

1. Simmer all your ingredients in a large pan for at least twenty minutes.

2. Use a strainer to pour your tea into a teapot or directly into mugs.

3. Add sweetness to taste!

Daily Goddesses

Many goddesses are associated with hearth and home, or elements like fire and food. May they help remind us that a kitchen is a place where magic can happen, where we can find joy and inspiration, not just the washing up!

Hestia (Greek) Goddess of hearth and home. Her name means hearth, fire and/or altar. Goddess Hestia reminds us that hearth and altar can be one and the same. She was the hearth fire burning in every home of ancient Greece. Sacred hearth fires were constantly tended within her temples and offerings of sweet wine and food made in her name. Despite this, Hestia isn't mentioned a lot in Greek mythology. And was (apparently) not considered particularly significant in Greek myth. She doesn't feature in Homer's *Odyssey*, and she is seldom represented in works of art. As the goddess of her own household, which would be Mount Olympus, she seldom leaves. So her presence in sweeping tales of mythology is small. She may well have been busy making supper, while other deities messed around with vengeance, smiting and seducing mortals.

I find this fascinating, in its mirror of homemaking in general. The kitchen witchery of cooking, cleaning and making a house a home often goes on quietly in the background of busy, noisy lives. To tend your hearth is not always a big and adventurous undertaking – but it is powerful and vital magic. So next time you are tending your home, allow yourself a little smile. Maybe light a candle and play music as you work. These tasks won't make the history books, but the magic of creating your home is precious. And in their own way, small acts of love, kindness and homemaking are the most exceptional magic of all. With these little doses of everyday magic, we are making life sweet and sacred for ourselves and others.

Maman Brigitte (Celtic + Voodoo) As one of our oldest, and many-faceted goddesses, Brigid has many roles and embodiments. As

I continue on my own path of training to be a Priestess of the Goddess Brigid, I am continually delighted to find new personifications of her around the world. Which brings us to Maman Brigitte: goddess of life, death, women, fertility, passion and healing. We will look at the Celtic version of Brigid in the Sun Magic chapter, but I felt she deserved an honourable mention within the kitchen realm, as in the Voodoo tradition she has a taste for rum infused with hot peppers. So you just know she's our kind of goddess! Should you connect to Maman Brigitte, you may well develop a taste for this fiery infusion as well. Brigitte arrived in the New World when women from Ireland were shipped to New Orleans to work as slaves and plantation workers. These women brought with them what little they could: tales of the goddess, particularly those that watched over women.

Like Brigid, Maman Brigitte was thought to be a healer. She was worshipped especially in times of needing healing or a fresh start. As goddess of the flame, Brigid in all her forms is associated with the hearth-fire. Where there is fire, there is Brigid. If you wanted to channel Maman Brigitte for a fresh start, a wee tot of rum and a chilli could be placed on your altar. Or, take a fiery swig of chilli infused rum, and breathe fire like a true goddess of power and passion!

Kerridwen (Celtic) Known as the 'Keeper of the Cauldron'; the cauldron would once have lived in the centre of the home, at the hearth. Kerridwen and her cauldron, are a symbol of knowledge and transformation. Working in the kitchen is the art of transformation. We take ingredients and transform them into something completely different, feeding ourselves and our families. You can celebrate Kerridwen every time you stir your supper. To draw in her powers, you can use some of the herbs and foods connected to her energy, try earthy bay leaf, nutmeg, sage, apples, pears and pumpkins.

Annapurna (Hindu) Goddess of food, kitchen and nourishment. Her name comes from *anna* meaning food and *purna* meaning filled. As goddess of nourishment, she never lets her devotees go hungry. Not only does the goddess provide nourishment to the body, but she also provides nourishment to the soul in the form of enlightenment, as she gives us the energy to attain knowledge. You can channel Annapurna as you reflect on all the things that nourish your body and your spirit: wholesome food, hot herbal teas, long baths, reading, singing, gardening, crafts, time with loved ones… Make time to nourish your soul as well as your body!

Closing Thoughts

Mother Earth really has provided magic in our food. Try as often as you can to eat food that is fresh and organic. Meals that you create yourself are infused with love that cannot be matched by ready-meals! Like any spell, cooking involves intuition and fun! Celebrate the magic you can create at your hearth and in your home.

See pictures of more recipes at **sentiayoga.com/yogaforwitches**

And don't forget to share your creations on Instagram with the hashtags #YogaforWitches and #YogaWitchCookBook

ANIMAL MAGIC

Numerous ancient mythologies and spiritual practices share a belief in the power of animals to guide and assist humans in their daily lives. Many of us would agree that animals are special and represent a link to nature that, as humans, we may wish to connect to.

In many cultures, animals have been and still are, revered, worshipped as spirits of nature, as power or spirit animals and animal guides of the gods. Animal behaviour can be a sign to what Mother Earth might be up to. One of the many reasons humans are particularly good at seeing patterns, symbols and meaning in almost anything is for its use to our survival. It was no less than life or death to recognise that migrating birds meant early snowfall or that flattened grasses meant a predator was near.

People have sought to bring animals into their magical practice and superstitions throughout the ages. There is a broad scope available to us as to how we may wish to connect to animals. We may use them as inspiration or to seek strength, we may want to call an animal to us or reflect on an animal's presence. While some may have animal companions for life, other animals may fly into your life just long enough to deliver a message. They may teach us something about our ability and strength or something that we need to pay attention to. And this

Familiars

A witch may choose certain animals as their link to nature, spirits and deities. Or in some way, find that an animal 'chooses' them. We can perform rituals and make offerings to their spirits in attempts to communicate, connect or in some way, gain insight.

The idea of the witches 'familiar' has suffered some of the same negative stereotypes as the witch herself. Presented sometimes as a demon attending to a witch or just as a spirit embodied in an animal to accompany, serve or guard as a close friend or associate. Anyone who owns a pet may well think of them as a friend or guardian of some kind. You may consider your pets your familiars, or not.

may be an encounter by day, by dreams or other symbols. Animals can walk alongside us as teachers, messengers and guides, helping us to better understand the world in which we live.

Power Animals

In some traditions of modern paganism and witchcraft, animal symbolism and parts of animals, such as feathers are incorporated into magical belief and practice. You may connect to the idea of having a familiar or channelling animal energy. Or you may wish to work with spirit, totem or power animals.

Shamans around the world believe that all beings, particularly animals, have a spirit or soul, and seek to relate to this spirit. Their ceremonies may involve dressing in animal furs, feathers, horns while performing dances and imitating the animal to attract parts of an animal's spirit and powers by mimicry.

Many cultures have a version of the power animal, spirit animal and spirit guide, though they are often associated with Native American cultures. The origin of the animal-inspired yoga poses are native to Asia. You will see animal correspondence associated with deities, often that share an element of their archetype. Such as the hound with huntress Diana and the wise owl with Minerva, goddess of wisdom. As you may imagine, the animals were most likely those native to the culture of the deity.

If you take time to learn about the symbolism of animals in different cultures, you may end up learning something new about yourself and your path. As always when exploring the cultures of others use humility and respect. This is not an invitation to appropriate (although I think it's misappropriation that is more the issue), but rather to appreciate and enjoy learning about the wildlife of other cultures too.

When reflecting on your power animals, I strongly recommend looking first to those native to your own cultural heritage, by engaging with your local natural wildlife and landscape. With this in mind, the animals I have outlined here are mainly European.

Meeting your Power Animal

In shamanic practice, one meets their power animal through meditation or a vision quest. If you'd like to draw a familiar or power animal to you, you can do this by meditation. Find a place to relax and allow your mind to become calm. You may imagine walking through a forest or an area of natural beauty where animals live. Focus your intent on meeting an animal companion, and see if you come into contact with any.

Animal Symbolism

Here are just some examples of what animals can symbolise and their appearance in cultures' myths throughout history. It may be that you encounter these animals in real life or wish to channel their energy. If you see animals in nature or feel particularly drawn to certain animals there may be messages and meaning you can explore. You will need to use your own intuition in determining what messages a particular animal may be trying to bring into your life, or why you are drawn to specific animal connections.

Hawk: Hawks may be a sign that you need to look at something more closely before proceeding. An influential lesson may be about to unfold.

Eagle: The eagle can remind us to be courageous and seek new heights. Tough choices may be on their way, but you are capable of more than you may think.

Raven/Crow: Seeing a crow or raven could mean that you are ready to let go of something or enter into a cycle of transformation. Crows are symbols of strength and creation – they call us to recognise the magic alive in the world.

Owl: An indicator that you need to pay attention to your intuition and wisdom and a sign to connect to your authentic self.

Lizard: May be a sign you need to pay attention to your goals, a reminder of your powers and abilities. Perhaps you have lost sight of what you are capable of.

Snake: The snake is a symbol of life force and passion. It could be that you need to attend to your desires and put energy into pursuing them. The snake may also suggest that you are entering into, or in need of, a time of healing and renewal.

Spider: Spiders are symbols of creativity and spiritual connectedness – an encouragement to tune into creative inspiration and to take time to create.

Dragonfly: Dragonflies can be a sign of spiritual journeying and an indication that you are making progress in the right direction. Once, while I was teaching a yoga class in large event room in a local hotel, a dragonfly appeared from nowhere and for a few minutes he flew around the ceiling, occasionally skimming though the chandeliers making delightful tinkling sounds. The yoga students were delighted!

Butterfly: A symbol of the power of transformation and growth. If you repeatedly see butterflies, it may be a sign that you need to release thoughts or feelings that are holding you back.

Wolf: The wolf may suggest looking to your 'pack', the people you are surrounding yourself with. It may be time to unite and reconnect with your family and loved ones. Or to accept help that is offered when you face challenges.

Fox: Foxes can suggest the need to adjust your thinking about something or the way you are approaching things. Foxes may also come as a joyful reminder not to take things too seriously.

Cat: The cat is representative of intuition and heart. Cats have magical associations, and are connected with powerful and wise goddesses like Bastet and Freya, as well as being eternally linked to witches!

Myth, Magic and Folklore

The following are just some of the animals woven into European and Norse folklore and an indication of the ideas they can represent. As with our tables of correspondence, every animal can signify many things, and these meanings can vary from person to person.

Ravens and Crows in Mythology

Common birds in European mythology, as they are numerous in these lands – ravens and crows clad in black plumage can be seen as ominous. In Shakespeare's *Macbeth*, both witches and ravens foretell imminent deaths…

(In Celtic mythology, there is a warrior goddess known as the Morrigan. She appears in the form of crows and ravens or is accompanied by a group of them. These birds are seen as a sign that the Morrigan is near.

(In the Norse pantheon, the God Odin is represented or accompanied by a pair of ravens: Huginn and Muinnin, names that translate as "thought" and "memory". These ravens bring Odin news each night from Midgard.

(For ancient Greeks, the crow is a symbol of Apollo, God of prophecy. Augury was the divination practice of using birds' behaviour as a guide: crows flying from the east or south was considered a good sign.

Rabbits in Folklore

In Europe, rabbits and hares are viewed as fertility symbols. Rabbits are nocturnal most of the year, but in March when mating season begins, they come out to frolic in the fields!

Rabbit Magic

☾ The well-known rabbit's foot charm can be good luck to those who carry it, although not suitable for vegans, or any animal lover. I prefer a metal or ceramic rabbit charm, the ones depicting the rabbit or hare staring at the moon are particularly beautiful and also help channel the boundless energy of rabbits and hares.

☾ If wild rabbits live in your garden, leave them offerings of lettuce or carrots.

☾ Rabbits and hares can go to ground quickly if in danger. You may wish to add rabbit hairs to a witch bottle for protection magic.

☾ In some cultures, rabbits and hares are considered messengers of the underworld, as they weave in and out of their earthy tunnels. If you're doing a meditation that involves an underworld journey such as connecting to ancestors or roots, you can call upon the rabbit to be your guide.

Wolves in Folklore

The wolf can capture people's imagination in both its beauty and power, it is a wild, untamed spirit. The wolf can fascinate, frighten, and draw us in. You'll find the wolf in many myths and legends from many North American and European cultures.

☾ In Scotland, the Cailleach is a crone goddess who brings forth the winter and dark half of the year. She is also portrayed riding a wolf and as a protector of wild things.

☾ For Romans, the wolf is responsible for no less than the founding of Rome…and an entire empire. The story of Romulus and Remus tells of orphaned infant twins who were saved from starvation and raised by a she-wolf. In some cultures, the wolf is still seen as a symbol of sovereignty and leadership. Where I live in Somerset, a small but beautiful statue of Romulus, Remus and the She-wolf looks down over commuters on the edge of the A36 near Wells. It was built with love by an Italian prisoner of war.

Bees in Folklore

Bees feature in folklore from many cultures. These are some of the legends:

☾ In Ancient Egypt, the honeybee was the royal symbol, used by pharaohs.

☾ The priestesses in Temples of Goddess Aphrodite were known as *melissae*, which means bees, and Aphrodite herself was called Melissa, the queen bee. You will still find melissae tending the Goddess temples in places such as Glastonbury and Bristol in the UK.

☾ In Celtic mythology, the bee is a wise messenger between our world and the spirit realm.

☾ Bees and honey are referenced in Hindu cultures and feature in the ancient texts of the Vedas. Honey was considered the food of the gods, able to banish evil spirits and carry the energy of life.

☾ Bees and honey appear in the Norse *Eddas* (literary works of myth and legend), often connected with Yggdrasil, the World Tree.

☾ Within the Witchcraft Museum in Boscastle, UK, you'll find an old folk charm that was found in Dawlish, that features three dead bumblebees in a bag. They look a little sad now, but it was believed to be a charm for health and happiness.

Animal Asana

Early yogis developed their practice deeply influenced by the world around them, as everything in nature offers something for humans to learn from. Hence, we have yoga poses inspired by animals, plants and elements. There are many yoga poses named after our animal friends. This menagerie of yoga poses includes: Cow, Camel, Cat, Dog, Lion, Monkey, Eagle, Peacock, Crow, Crane, Pigeon, Cobra, Crocodile, Tortoise, Locust, Scorpion, Firefly and Grasshopper.

As we journey through yoga to unite the body, mind, and spirit, animals are a fantastic inspiration: strong, agile, flexible, instinctive and aware. Animal poses are a connection with aspects of the environment that we often forget in our busy lives. It is a beautiful thing to learn the mythology behind yoga poses and embody a little of that myth and magic in the pose.

*If you wish to practice some of these poses, I suggest seeking out a class and teacher. To see images of these poses and explore them in more detail head to **sentiayoga.com/yogaforwitches***

Cobra Pose – Bhujangasana

Snakes hold an honoured place in Hindu mythology. Some Hindu myths say the earth itself is supported upon a coiled snake, known as Ananta, meaning 'The Endless'. You may also have made this connection between yoga and snakes from earlier in this book, where we looked at kundalini energy, often envisaged as a coiled snake at the bottom of your spine. As snakes shed their skins, they represent the idea of regeneration, transformation and renewal. Always to be treated with great respect, the snake is also destroyer. In embedding the energy of the snake in this pose, we rise a little higher towards enlightenment.

Bhujanga means 'serpent' in Sanskrit, in our cobra pose we are the serpent rising to strike, strong and powerful. Laying on your belly, place your palms on the floor under your shoulders, fingertips pointing forwards. Hug your elbows to your sides. Press your hands into the floor and begin to lift your chest, engage the muscles of your centre to support you as you rise. Keep your thighs firmly rooted in the earth. Allow your gaze and heart to expand to the sky. You can use your hands as support, but you are lifting from your core. Keep your elbows soft and shoulders relaxed.

Cow Pose – Bitilasana – and Cat Pose – Marjaryasana

Cows are sacred in Hindu mythology, and feature heavily in myths; the cow is seen as an embodiment of Lakshmi, the goddess of wealth. Prithvi, the goddess of the earth, regularly uses this form as well.

Cats are a little rarer in Hindu stories. However, the goddess Shashthi, the protectress of children, is often portrayed riding a cat or with a cat face.

The gentle flex and flow of Cow and Cat starts with a flat back, kneeling on all fours. From here we flex inwards with the spine in Cow Pose, raising head and tailbone and flex outwards with rounded spine in Cat Pose, dropping the head and tailbone. Moving with the breath, these two poses flow together to create a rhythmic movement in tune with the breath.

Cow Face Pose – Gomukhasana

My favourite myth/origin story around this pose is that when the goddess Ganga (who would become the River Ganges) fell to earth, she landed in the Himalayas and formed a glacier. The glacier's peaks resembled a cow's head, and the source of the Ganges river flows from it. This glacier opening is called Gaumukh – 'the cow's mouth' – combining perfectly the ideas of the cow, water and goddess as life-giving mothers.

From seated, bend your knees and put your soles on the earth. Bring your left foot under the right knee to the outer right hip. Cross your right leg over the left, stacking the right knee on top of the left, the right foot comes to the outside of the left hip. The shape of your legs is intended to represent the cow, your stacked knees are the nose and your feet are the ears! Sit evenly on the sitting bones. From here you can bring in cow face arms (one elbow points to the sky, the other to the earth, hands clasped behind the back), or just work with sitting in this way for a few breaths.

Lion Pose – Simhasana

Lion Pose assumes the sitting position and facial expression of a lion. From the Sanskrit word for lion, *simha*, this pose evokes the energy and roar of this powerful animal. The pose combines both asana (physical posture) and pranayama (breath work) to produce a deep roaring exhalation during the peak of Lion Pose. It's also a great pose to release anger and have a bit of a giggle! (I defy anyone to do this pose without ending up smiling!)

From an easy cross-legged seat or sitting back on the heels, place your hands on your knees. As you exhale deeply, spread your paws (fingers) wide, open your mouth wide, stick your tongue out and gaze to the sky. The exhale should be audible as you roar. On the inhale, bring your face back to neutral, relaxing the neck, chest, and hands. Roar and repeat!

Animal Goddesses

Many goddesses have associated animals, and some are patronesses of animal care. A few were most often depicted *as* animals.

Eingana (Australian Aboriginal) Also known as the "Dreamtime Snake" as she resides within the dreams of humans. She is creatrix and mother to all the living things of the earth. Also found in similar forms in Greece and India, serpent goddesses symbolise life, energy, healing, and movement between the spirit worlds.

Bastet (Egyptian) The cat goddess of wisdom, independence and strength, she carries with her the energy of balance and protection. Graceful, independent, playful, and intuitive, Bastet casts a watchful eye over the world, seeking justice and equality. Bastet is a rarity in being the goddess of both moon and sun; in this way she represents yin and yang, and is a great reminder to seek balance. She is a wonderful goddess to work with when you are seeking a rebalancing of power or reclaiming of your own power.

Kamadhenu (Hindu) Divine bovine-goddess, the miraculous "cow of plenty" and the "mother of cows" represented all cows; and the source of prosperity they signify in Hindu culture. She featured in the Vedas, and apparently is quite fond of granting wishes! The cow is also found in many tribes in Africa, representing all things life and vitality.

Closing Thoughts

A dog does not worry how it looks as it stretches after a nap, it just moves in a way that feels good. Birds do not feel self-conscious about dancing for their mate. And lions do not hold back from a battle, fearing they are not strong enough. Each animal follows its instincts with complete trust in its purpose and abilities. So when you next practice yoga, ritual or spell, think about how unburdened by worry, shame or indecision animals embody their power completely. Once you let your mind quieten and release the thoughts that can complicate and cloud our intuition, you may find greater power and simplicity in your practice. Discover and connect to your animal guides, find out what they symbolise in your life and learn how animal magic can help you navigate your life on earth.

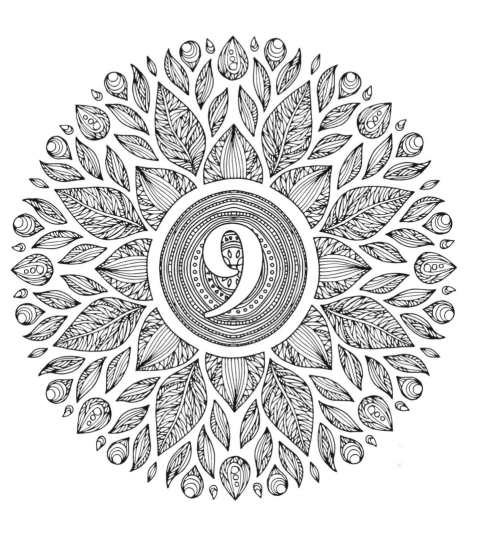

MOON MAGIC

The moon is our closest celestial neighbour. Our ancestors would have gazed up at its silvery glow and tried to make sense of its rhythms, using the changing faces of the moon to chart the months and seasons. Many humans feel a connection to earth's beautiful natural satellite. The rhythms of the planet are ever moving: years, seasons, weeks, days. These many spirals have a magic all of their own – and one you can connect to, should you choose.

Moon Magic for Witches

The moon represents many things to the witch: goddess, divine feminine, feminine power and cycles of energy. You may well have heard the term 'drawing down the moon' which is an essential ritual in many pagan and witch traditions, where the spirit of the Goddess is invoked. Harnessing the power of each moon phase can help connect with your strengths. And makes for some beautiful spells and rituals.

Many witches connect to the cycle of the waxings and wanings of the moon, each having their own special energy. A little lunar knowledge can help to harness the energy of each moon phase if you want to call upon it. So, with this in mind, here are some ideas for magic based upon various lunar stages.

Moon Phases

Many simple free apps will tell you what the moon phase is right now, and many diaries and calendars have the details printed in as well. Each moon phase, though constantly changing, is in such tiny increments that to our naked eye may appear to last up to three days and the lunar cycle does not match up exactly with the calendar month; it's about 29 days (which is why sometimes we have a month with two full moons!)

The main moon phases are: new, waxing crescent, first quarter, waxing gibbous, full, waning gibbous, last quarter, waning crescent,

Drawing Down the Moon

There are many ways to draw down the moon, and the methods vary, depending on your needs and tradition. This is a simple version you can do standing at your altar or outside under the full moon.

Call the Goddess:

Mother Goddess of the moon.
Lend me your guiding light
Please shine upon my work this night.

Raise your arms to the sky to greet the Goddess/moon:

I am Goddess. I am earth, air, ether, water and fire,
I am stone, wind, ocean, magic and pyre,
You may call upon me always.
May you find my beauty, strength, wisdom, within you.

Take a few moments to absorb the full moon's glow. From here you may wish to cast a full moon spell (such as a spell for growth) draw oracle cards, or simply meditate.

and balsamic. Though there are some specific ideas about what magic can be worked at each phase, listening to your own intuition and cycles is always a good idea.

New Moon

The night sky is at its darkest at the new moon. For around three days during each lunar cycle, after the moon has waned, just a ghost of an outline can be seen in the sky. New moons are new beginnings, a fresh start. The new moon is a beautiful time to set goals and intentions for the forthcoming cycle, and reflect on what you hope to achieve. What do you want the coming month to look like? Is there a joyless job that you're finally ready to leave to make room for the career of your dreams? The new moon is a time to encourage beginnings and let go of the past. A time to turn inwards and replenish, a perfect time for yoga nidra, meditation and journaling.

The dark skies of the new moon can be the best phase for rest and reflection; you may not want to actively practice any magic or yoga, and that's okay. This can be a chance to give yourself a break, to turn inwards and replenish. Meditation and reflection can be useful, though, as you explore questions, emotions or concerns that require time for you to process. Plant seeds of intentions and watch them grow as the moon grows brighter in the sky through the month.

Magical moon practices for harnessing new moon energy include:

☾ Cleansing and purifying the body and mind (See the New Moon Bath Ritual below).

☾ Simple magic related to inner harmony and peace – like drinking chamomile tea.

☾ Mindfulness and meditation.

☾ Getting in touch with your inner self, reaffirming personal and spiritual goals – you may want to journal, free write, paint, collage your goals – whatever works to help you connect.

☾ Write down anything you wish to let go of in this new lunar cycle and throw it into Kerridwen's cauldron; you may just scrunch up the note and throw into a pot or burn (carefully!) your paper in a cauldron if you have one.

New Moon Bath Ritual

I love bringing a little magic and ritual to activities already in my schedule. Spells can be intricate and elaborate, but they don't have to be. They can be as simple and delightful as enjoying a cleansing bath on a new moon.

I am particularly fond of a little bath magic. After all, why not make use of the giant cauldron we have in our bathrooms! Run yourself a hot bath and pour in some cleansing salts such as Epsom salts or Himalayan pink salt. Add some dried chamomile or passionflower to the bath to help soothe and calm, perhaps some rose petals to add love and release anger. You can buy both in bulk online, tie them in a muslin bag if you wish or let them float around the tub!

Light a candle if you wish. You can channel simple candle magic with a white candle for cleansing or blue for contemplation. As you relax in the bath, visualise the past soaking off you: hurts, bad habits and grudges, anything you want to let go of. If it helps you can write them down, focusing the energy and feelings you have as you write. You can write something like "I release self-doubt" or "I am done with hating my body". When you eventually get out, all these things can go down the drain (the notes can be burnt or thrown away with intention).

Waxing Moon

The moon is increasing in illumination; the journey from new to full takes around fourteen days as it passes through the waxing crescent, first quarter moon and waxing gibbous phases. We may feel a little more extroverted or action-oriented in our energy; this is the perfect time to take action. You can use this time to perform magic to manifest and attract positive energy and intentions. The waxing moon is 'phase two' of your intention rituals as you take actions towards your new moon goals.

☾   A spell for abundance or money.

☾ A visualisation of getting a new job or home.

☾ Manifestation rituals.

☾ Vision boards.

Waxing Crescent – Time to begin exploring your dreams, exploring how you might move forward and create your path.

First Quarter – The first quarter moon marks the halfway point between the new moon and the approaching full moon. Like the equinoxes, quarter moons are a time for intentional action and preparation as we tip over into a new phase.

Waxing Gibbous – As we continue our journey to fullness, gather and hold momentum in your actions. As the moon's light grows and blooms, so do your personal goals.

Full Moon

This lunar stage has the potential for great power. Whilst the moon generally represents a calming energy, now it is reflecting the full light of the sun: a more heightened, dynamic energy is occurring. Just as the full moon draws the tides higher, it can also heighten our emotions. Depending on how you are already feeling you may feel more positive or more hopeful, or you might feel more anger or frustration. Try and bear that in mind if you are feeling emotions strongly over a full moon.

The full moon is a chance to be thankful for everything we have: a time of growth and gratitude. The bright light of the full moon can illuminate elements of our lives. And this can feel good if our plans are coming into fruition or challenging if that extra light is highlighting cracks in relationships or arrangements. And sometimes, in the light of the full moon, I feel a bit like a rabbit in the headlights and just freeze. So it is okay if you don't feel like doing anything at full moon. But, if you do want to harness this powerful energy with spell work, this is an excellent time to do rituals addressing personal and spiritual growth.

☾ Spells related to increasing your intuition and awareness.

☾ Rituals that connect you with the goddess, such as 'drawing down the moon'.

☾ Any magic related to developing your skills (this can be as simple as reading a book, or maybe practising reading tarot, pendulum work or scrying).

☾ Moon bathe: absorb the moonbeams from a safe space outside, or by a window. (Often witches will cleanse crystals or jewellery in the light of the full moon).

Divination

Divination is the art and craft of foretelling the future and uncovering secrets. Like magic, forms of divination have existed (and continue to exist) in all cultures, as we have sought through the centuries to see what fate has in store for us and our ventures. Reading omens and communicating with other realms can be done by methods including, but not limited to: pendulum work, scrying, reading tarot, tea leaves and crystal balls. Divination using the moon specifically is called selenomancy named for the ancient Greek moon goddess Selene.

A friend of mine even once met an asparamancer – who used asparagus to predict the future!

Fear surrounding these practices, like witchcraft, has developed from organised religion and fearful factions branding occult practices such as divination evil or harmful. Many people, while accepting that there are no certainties, find hope, empowerment and inspiration in the practice.

Waning Moon

As the waning moon journeys from full to new moon once more, its light decreases. This can be a time of the month to do magic that casts away, or lets go of anything you no longer wish to hold onto, so that you can start anew with the next new moon. The waning moon is the time for slowing down and reflecting. You are readying yourself for the next new moon to set an intention and to leap into action in the next waxing period.

☾ Rituals to cut negative people or relationships from your life.

☾ Rituals to release bad habits or energy.

☾ Meditations to release anything that no longer serves you.

☾ Magic related to reducing things, such as fear or illness.

Waning Gibbous – Release and regroup. Reflect on and accept what you have discovered on your journey thus far.

Last Quarter – Once more moving towards balance, perhaps it's time to let go in some way.

Waning Crescent – You may want to reflect on the steps you wish to take next. Review and learn what you can from your mistakes.

Balsamic Moon – A few days before the new moon, the moon goes 'balsamic,' which is the very last little sliver of the waning moon before it disappears from view and goes dark.

As you wind down and complete a month-long lunar cycle, the balsamic moon reminds you to let go of draining commitments, toxic relationships, and anything else that does not serve you.

Moon Spells

Correspondences associated with the moon can be helpful when creating a spell or setting up an altar. If you want to perform a candle spell, for instance, it's nice to know colours associated with the moon. If you're going to anoint the candle, or burn incense, then you can use associated herbs.

☾ *Colours: silver, blue, black, white, purple.*

☾ *Oils: jasmine, cypress, clary sage, rosemary, lavender.*

☾ *Animals: wolf, owl, bat, rabbit, moth.*

☾ *Herbs and plants: jasmine, moonflower, moonwort, sage, cypress, lavender (especially white lavender).*

Esbats: Moon Festivals

Esbats are celebrations of the thirteen full moons that occur every year. The word *Esbat* can refer to any ritual that honours the Goddess in her association with the moon. When the full moon lights up the night sky, witches may honour the Goddess. And many covens may come together to hold rituals and work magic at this time.

Not every witch celebrates the full moon. Some witches and covens choose to meet at the new moon, the beginning of the lunar cycle: new moon is when I head to Glastonbury for new moon ceremonies with the priestesses of Kerridwen.

Moon Magic for Yogis

In yoga, you'll often hear references to the moon, whether that's in the name of a pose (e.g. Half Moon and Crescent Moon pose) the moon phase or teachings of yoga philosophy. For example, I often mention it to the class if I am teaching on the day of a new moon or full moon. It can be a helpful, energetic theme for the day's yoga practice, i.e. introspection during a new moon, gratitude for the full moon.

Why is the moon significant in yoga? And how it can help deepen your practice and connection with the earth?

Well, it starts with the name...

Hatha yoga is the term used to describe the practice of combining physical postures of yoga asana and pranayama. Hatha probably describes most accurately the yoga we now practice in the West.

Hatha yoga, as outlined in such texts as the *Hatha Yoga Pradipika*, has a greater focus on the physical body, and what to do with it, than Patanjali's original outline. In Sanskrit, *ha* is a seed sound that relates to the masculine dynamic energy of the sun and *tha* to the feminine intuitive moon. Together, they relate to the balance of masculine and feminine energy within us all. When combined, the word *hatha* means "energy" or "force" in Sanskrit: hatha is a determined effort to bring our dual nature into balance.

In Patanjali's *Yoga Sutras*, the universe is described as being made up of male (*purusha*) and female (*prakriti*) energy. Other deities/energies are mentioned in different yoga styles such as in Tantra yoga: the male is *Shiva* and female *Shakti*. So there is always this interplay between male and female, yang and yin, divine masculine and the divine feminine, sun and moon. The sun is our masculine energy – energetic and active, and the moon is feminine energy – calm and grounded. When we practice yoga, we are working toward uniting these masculine and feminine energies. A typical Hatha yoga class might move from energising poses like Sun Salutations, onto calming poses, before meditation and relaxation.

Guru Purnima

*On the day of the full moon (*purnima *is a Sanskrit word for full moon) in the Hindu month of* Ashad *(July–August) a festival called Guru Purnima is observed: a Hindu tradition dedicated to spiritual and academic teachers, and their sharing of this wisdom. Traditionally celebrated by Hindus and Buddhists, it is a time to honour teachers and guides who have helped you on your path and spiritual journey. In some religions, gurus are regarded as a link between the individual and the divine. For many Hindus, Guru Purnima is a time to honour these great gurus and spend time in group reflection (known as* satsang*).*

I encourage students to use Guru Purnima to reconnect with their own sources of inspiration and learning. Your gurus may be ancestors, family, friends, people who have inspired and awakened something in you. Your gurus may also be found in the natural world, maybe you find inspiration amongst animals and trees. You may wish to acknowledge your teachers on Guru Purnima or any full moon.

New Moon and Full Moon for Yogis

Many yogis believe we are physically as well as energetically affected by the phases of the moon. The moon can influence the kind of yoga we practice or feel like practising. Or in some cases, the desire not to practice at all. Indeed, in some yoga traditions, full moon and new moon days are yoga holidays. Practising yoga over time can help us attune to these natural cycles. And you can decide for yourself whether to practice yoga in line with the lunar cycles or not.

Both sun and moon apply an influence upon the earth. The differences of energies during a new and full moon have been compared to the rise and fall of breath and energy in the body. Known in yoga as *prana* and *apana*: prana governs the 'drawing in' of breath, while apana is the 'letting go'. The full moon mirrors the top of an inhalation; a peak of energy builds in the body. You may feel this yourself as you inhale and hold your breath. During the full moon, we tend to be more dynamic and more likely to take action. And at new moon, we release, like the letting go of apana. Deeply exhale. Notice as your lungs empty, muscles relax and your energy naturally drains away with the breath, moving towards stillness. During the new moon, our energy may be more contemplative.

New moon for yogis is an excellent time to practice yin and restorative yoga and generally take it easy. During full moon is a powerful time to take action, practising an energetic yoga class, like Hatha or Vinyasa yoga, and embracing your yang energy.

Moon Salutation

Chandra Namaskara is a flowing yoga sequence which honours the moon. The Sanskrit word *chandra* means "moon" and *namaskara* "salutation" from *namas*, which means "to bow to" (The phrase we use to close our yoga classes, *namaste*, also comes from this root.) Chandra Namaskara is a cooling, meditative sequence of postures, which is ideal to be practised in the evening. These postures can also be used in the same practice as Sun Salutation to balance their dynamic energy and embrace both sun and moon.

The sequence of asana in Chandra Namaskara has many variations, but will often involve moving from one side of the mat to the other. The side stretches and movements of the sequence signify the phases of the moon as it waxes and wanes.

Like many yoga asana, Chandra Namaskara is a recent yogic creation, but practices of worshipping the moon are ancient. Just as witchcraft techniques and practices may have changed in modern times, it all started with awe and respect for the heavenly bodies above us; yogis and witches have both gazed up at the moon and felt magic in their hearts. Drawing on moon energy can help illuminate a path of comfort and joy, to help you find your way on the darkest of nights.

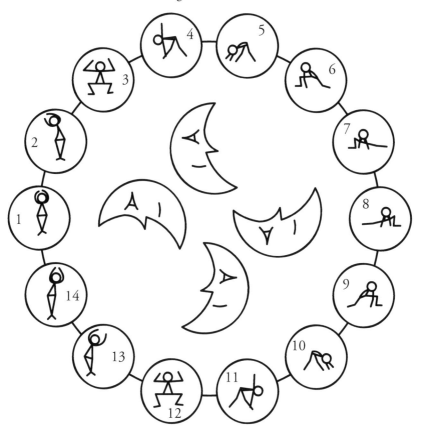

Moon Salutation Sequence

Hold in your mind the idea that as you travel from one side of your mat to the other, you are tracing the journey of the moon through the night sky:

☾ Upward Salute – palms together overhead.

☾ Crescent Moon Pose – arching to the left.

☾ Goddess Pose – a wide squat stance, arms like a cactus, palms forward. (A similar power stance to the Haka!)

☾ Triangle Pose – extending to the left, right arm up.

☾ Pyramid Pose – to left leg.

(Lunge to the left.

(Forward Facing Lunge – right leg extended.

(Travel through Squat Pose – Malasana.

(Forward Facing Lunge – left leg extended.

(Lunge to the right.

(Head to Knee – right leg.

(Triangle Pose – extending to the right, left arm up.

(Goddess Pose.

(Crescent Moon Pose – arching to the right.

(Return to Upward Salute – palms together overhead.

To learn more about practising Moon Salutations, and to see video sequences of the Sun, Moon and Earth sequences, check out my resource page **sentiayoga.com/yogaforwitches**

Moon Goddesses

Channelling goddess energy can be of powerful use to witches and yogis alike. Many of the lunar goddesses such as Hecate and Kerridwen, are also connected with magic and the intuitive nature of women. Working with the moon is to honour your sensitivity, rather than seeing it as a weakness. The goddesses can guide us through dark nights, with their lanterns filled with soft moonlight.

Arianrhod (Celtic) This Celtic goddess of the moon and stars, has palaces both in the heavens and on earth – Caer Arianrhod, a resting place for souls, is the constellation also known as the Corona Borealis. And on earth, Caer Arianrhod takes the form of submerged rocks and reefs off the coast of northern Wales. Her name means "silver wheel", representing the Wheel of the Year, fate and destiny, the spinning wheel weaving the tapestry of our lives.

Hina (Hawaiian) Hina started life as a mortal woman but grew weary of the noises and stresses of the earth. She retreated to the moon to find peace and calm (I think we can all relate to that!) From her moon perch, she helps guide sailors across the ocean. You may not be able to retreat to the moon, but find a retreat space today, even if it is just for five minutes. A yoga class, a meditation in a quiet room, a cup of tea in a cosy chair: channel Hina as you take time for yourself so that you can help others when they need you.

Closing Thoughts

Whatever phase the moon is in, observing it in the night sky can be a reminder to pause, to create quiet space for yourself for contemplation and self-reflection. Taking time to acknowledge or reflect on the moon is an acknowledgement of the cycles we embody and live within – a lunar reminder to listen to your intuition.

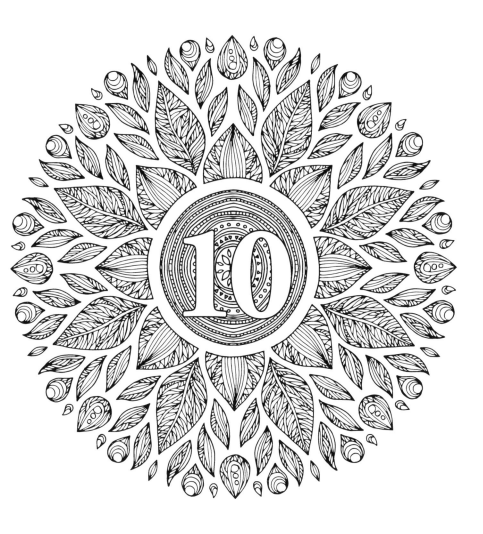

SUN MAGIC

We have explored the popularity of the moon in the previous chapter. We see the symbols of the sun a little less often in witchcraft, perhaps because the sun, to many, represents masculine energy, and the moon connects more with the intuitive work that much of magic embodies. However, the sun's energy and solar cycles can be powerful and splendid energies to work with. And, as we'll see, the sun can also represent the divine feminine. We can harness the energy of sunrise, noon and sunset in a similar way to the lunar cycles: sunrise is a great time to address matters like new beginnings, inspiration and love, whereas sunset is ideal for things like releasing.

Daily Cycle of the Sun

Sunrise

As both we and the sun rise in the morning, it's a great time to do a ritual and start your day with magic. The light of the morning sun will come from the east, which you can use as a focal point to attune to the sun and earth. As you start your new day, you may imagine the sun's rays blasting away any negative energies, leaving you ready to start a beautiful new day.

Midday

The sun is at its highest point in the sky and highest level of energy at midday. You may use the strength of the sun to help you overcome indecision or negativity. If you need guidance or inspiration, you can cast a spell, pitch a new idea or plan a new project under the light of this 'high point' of the day.

Sunset

Sunset is a special time, as the sun casts beautiful colours in the dimming light of the day. Dusk is a time of calmness and serenity. What can make sunset special is that it is a threshold, between day and night, between two worlds. This is when many witches find a special time for magic. If you feel a need to transition, or start something new or let go of something, this is the perfect time to hold a ritual. This could be a good time to communicate with spirit guides or ancestors and call upon them for guidance or wisdom.

Sun Magic for Witches

☾ Make lemon tea. Those little slices of lemon are like little bursts of sunshine! To the Kitchen Witch, the lemon has associations with sun, cleansing, happiness, hope, and love. Make lemon tea and either drink or pour it near the roots of a tree and make a wish. Or add dried slices of lemon or orange to your altar as an offering.

☾ Create a sun altar. Choose a spot with plenty of natural light, such as a windowsill. Place fire and sun elements on your altar, these might include: incense to burn, golden coins, yellow candles, fire agate, carnelian and amber. You may also want to arrange your items in a mandala or sun shape.

☾ Grow plants and flowers. Spending time in the sun to tend flowers is a beautiful way to connect to the sun's energy. Whether you have a garden, balcony or a windowsill. Channel your inner Green Witch and give some time and love to help plants bloom!

☾ Make a sun jar. Fill a jar (preferably glass) with water and set it in a bright spot to absorb the light of sunbeams. You can include other items associated with the sun: a piece of carnelian, a drop of lemon essential oil, lemon slices or a handful of sunflower or marigold petals. Place this jar your altar as a symbol of the sun, or use as an additional energy boost in your next bath!

Sun Spells

Correspondences associated with the sun can be helpful when creating a spell or setting up an altar. If you want to perform a candle spell, for instance, it's nice to know colours associated with the sun. If you're going to anoint the candle, or burn incense, then you can use associated herbs.

☾ *Colours: gold, orange, amber, yellow, red.*

☾ *Oils: orange, cinnamon, frankincense, lemon, clove.*

☾ *Animals: lion and hawk.*

☾ *Herbs and plants: sunflower, marigold, dandelion, orange, lemon, saffron, buttercup, daisy, cloves, cinnamon.*

Energy Magic

The sun has both nourishing and healing properties. If you are feeling tired, the sun can give you a boost of energy to help energise and brighten your day.

Go outside where you can bathe in sunlight and feel the rays shining over you. Feel the energy from the sun radiate down from the top of your head, through your body, travelling down your spine, into your arms and legs, to the very tips of your fingers and toes. Visualise that you are glowing with golden light from the inside out. Filled with sun fire, you emit a glow which creates a glowing shield around you. This shield can protect you, and you can draw energy from it.

It is lovely to perform this ritual outside, but if that's not possible, then find a sunny space in front of a window. On dull days you can light a candle, or make a hot drink. You may wish to call the directions or invoke a sun goddess or god. Close your eyes and focus on the sun, its warmth and light. Imagine the rays of light are wrapping around you in a hug. You may experience a feeling of heat and light; you may even receive words of wisdom or support. When you step out of the embrace, know that you have absorbed everything you need. When you go back inside, or into the shade, the energy of the sun is within you, healing your body, bringing you strength and comfort.

Sun Magic for Yogis

Light is a symbol of consciousness and illumination, and the sun is revered by ancient and modern yogis alike. Hindus consider the sun, called *surya* in Sanskrit, both the physical and spiritual centre of our universe and the creator of all life. One way to honour the sun for the yogi is through the dynamic sequence *Surya Namaskara* (Sun Salutation). In honouring the sun, we may also connect to our own inner fire. Sun Salutations can help us feel light and energised: perfect for morning practice.

Though there is disagreement over the origins of the Sun Salutation (this is a truth for every single yoga pose!), Namaskaras were first described in writing around 1500BCE in the *Rig Veda* (the oldest collection of the sacred Hindu scriptures). The rituals offered at sunrise and sunset were the bringing of the whole body to the earth and then rising again. Though they have changed a lot, the salutations we practice today mirror this ritual of release, connection and surrender.

I have no doubt that ancient yogis would have honoured the sun in some way, and numerous variations have evolved over the years. But one constant for me is that I always like to start and end in standing (Tadasana) with hands in prayer mudra at my heart as a chance to pause and reconnect to the breath. I often say to my students, "It is more important to feel the connection of movement and breath than to get the actual poses 'right'". So try and let go of concerns about 'doing it right' and try instead to find your 'flow' in the sequence.

Moving from posture to posture can be timed with your inhalation and exhalation. It is always useful to use long, calm breaths through your nose, as it gives you more time to move through the poses un-hurried! As you become more familiar with the sequence, you can start to really let the mind clear and just flow with the body and breath in a dance, almost, to greet the sun! Be mindful and unhurried with the poses, and be aware that the movements in between are just as important as the poses themselves.

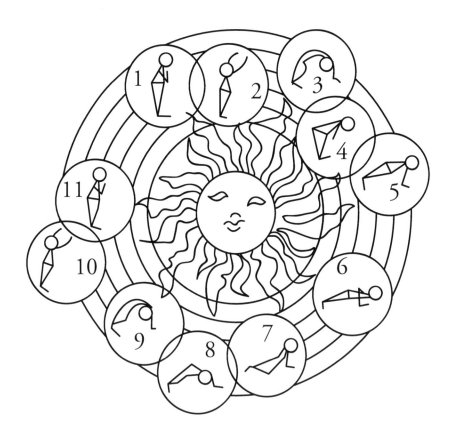

Sun Salutation Sequence

☾ Mountain Pose – with hands at heart.

☾ Upward Salute.

☾ Standing Forward Bend.

☾ Extend spine into a 'flat back'.

☾ Step back – (leading with right leg) into…

☾ High Plank Pose.

☾ Low Plank Pose.

☾ Cobra Pose.

☾ Downward-Facing Dog Pose.

☾ Step forward (leading with right leg) into…

☾ Standing Forward Bend.

☾ Upward Salute.

☾ Mountain Pose – with hands at heart.

☾ Repeat, leading with left leg.

If you can, it is a beautiful and special ritual to practice Sun Salutation outdoors, facing the east to the rising sun. But for many of us, that isn't possible! You could try doing a few rounds at the next equinox or solstice to acknowledge the change in the light. (In some yoga traditions, we practice 108 Sun Salutations to celebrate each solstice and equinox!)

A simple and lovely morning ritual can be a few rounds of Sun Salutations, and five minutes spent in meditation. And if you wish, a little time to reflect and journal before you start your day. (You can see more about journaling in Chapter 6.)

To see videos of Sun Salutations, head to my resource page for this book: **sentiayoga.com/yogaforwitches**

The Yoga Ritual of 108 Sun Salutations

Renowned mathematicians of Vedic culture viewed 108 as the number signifying the wholeness of existence. Traditionally, practising 108 Sun Salutations is reserved for the change of the seasons (the winter and summer solstice, and the spring and autumnal equinoxes).

Many yogis like to practice 108 Sun Salutations for the new year, and other significant life events. The heat that you build during this practice is cleansing and detoxifying. Heating the body and activating prana ignites a release of energy and emotions that no longer serve you. Within this yoga ritual is an invitation to surrender to the process, to find your flow, acknowledge any emotions that arise, and then let them go.

Sun Goddesses

Many solar deities are depicted as male, as it is common to represent the power of the moon with the divine feminine, and the energy of the sun with the divine masculine. However, the sun can be a feminine force, and there are some awesome solar goddesses lighting up the sky...

Sulis (Celtic) The goddess of sun and water is particularly close to my heart, as a resident of former Aquae Sulis (the Waters of Sulis) which is now Bath, UK. When they invaded, the Romans brought their own deities and beliefs with them to the predominantly Celtic and pagan lands of Somerset. Merging the goddess Minerva with her pagan counterpart, the Romans created a brand-new goddess for the city: Sulis Minerva. But Sulis is special in her own right: Sulis means sight or sun – and in yoga classes, I often relate her energy to the third eye chakra, which is the seat of our intuition. Sulis can help guide us to see things more clearly and illuminate our path. Being a water goddess as well, she can bless any ceremony or ritual with water or healing. Water is considered a feminine element and related to emotional healing.

Amaterasu (Japanese) Her name means 'great shining heaven' and her emblem, the rising sun, appears on the Japanese flag. According to legend, Amaterasu is responsible for keeping balance and harmony within the earthly realm. When you are feeling unbalanced, seek some time to channel Amaterasu by both grounding and absorbing the sun's light, get out in the garden, go for a walk, sit in the sun.

Áine (Celtic) This Irish goddess represents the spark of life; a sun goddess who is also the goddess of healing, love, fertility and prosperity. Often represented as a fairy queen as well as a goddess, Áine is a reminder of the radiance of summer and of the power love and joy to help us find light in the dark.

Sehkmet (Egyptian) This warrior goddess is depicted as a lioness, the fierce hunter. She represents both the power and the destructive qualities of the sun's rays, causing drought and famine. Sehkmet represents the awesome power of the sun; she is a wonderful goddess to work with to remind us of our own inner power, our own inner lioness, and embracing strength, even when it seems scary.

Brigid (Celtic) A Celtic fire goddess, Brigid is so ancient a deity she has countless incarnations as both goddess and saint, and is known by many names – Brigit, Bride, Bridghe, Saint Brigid and Brigantia. As a solar deity she is connected to light and elements of fire – health, hearth and home. Particularly around her festival, Imbolc on February 1st, you can call on Brigid's energy to find sparks of inspiration or relight the flames of forgotten dreams. Those training to be modern day priestesses of Brigid (like me!) learn of her energy in every season of the Wheel of the Year from Bridie the maiden at Imbolc to Brighid the Great Mother and crone at Samhain and Yule. And her animal correspondence; swan, snake, cow, wolf and the magical unicorn, selkie, phoenix and dragon.

Closing Thoughts

The sun is the active, dynamic yang energy to the moon's restorative, reflective yin energy. As with all things, balance is vital. Take time to rest and reflect, but there will be times when you must be brave and harness your inner fire, your sparks of passion and stride out into the world with all the power of the Goddess, magic and the sun within you!

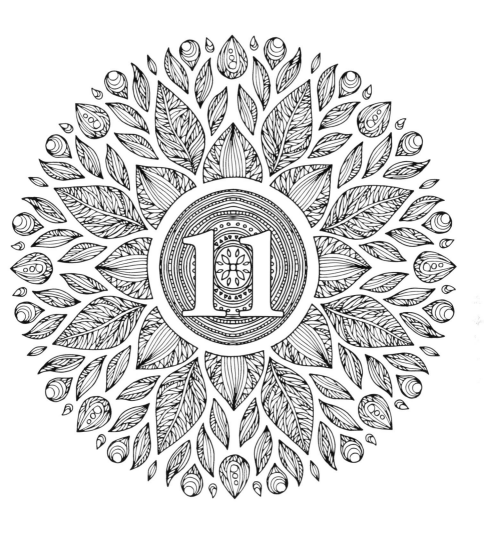

EARTH MAGIC

Often we can be so focused on what lies beyond us: the sun, moon and stars…we forget what lies beneath us: the earth. It can be a real challenge for us to act instinctively and naturally in the concrete man-made world, which is so unconnected to Mother Earth. So the simplest and fastest way to connect to earthly magic is to get outside onto and into the earth!

When you are out walking the earth, you can harness simple mindfulness practices. Take a pause to observe your senses, what you can see, feel, hear and smell. Ritual can be used to acknowledge the specialness of a moment, we do this with festivals and esbats, but you can do it on any day: they are all special after all.

I often find out in nature, I want to savour a particular moment. You can make your own wild altar in nature, gather twigs, leaves and fallen blossoms. Perhaps you may feel inspired to create a circle around yourself in leaves or pine cones…or mark the directions with acorns. Alternatively, you can forage for items to bring home to create an earth altar. These are particularly lovely in autumn and winter, seasons which are often linked in correspondence to the earth element. A simple earth altar can include stones, nuts, bones, and any pieces of nature you find – who doesn't love a shiny conker?

Sacred spaces are also splendid in gardens: hang up garlands of twigs and flowers, build fairy stacks of pebbles, make a mini stone circle. Go all-out if you wish and dedicate your whole garden to sacred earth magic!

Earth Magic

If you want to delve in deeper and sink your hands into the earth, there are many earth-related topics to explore, from magical to practical.

Ley lines: These are energy lines and alignments of many places of geographical interest, such as ancient monuments and megaliths.

Wildcrafting: Wildcrafting is harvesting plants from their natural habitat, usually for food and medicinal purposes.

Sacred Stones: There are stones that are considered sacred around the world. Some for their natural shape or formation, some because of what has been carved on them, and some which were arranged ritually by ancient humans. There are over a thousand stone circles in the British Isles, where I'm from, but you'll find sacred stones in every continent of the world.

Used in ancient times for ritual and ceremony, they are wonderful places to visit to connect to ancient earth energy. If you have never been to a stone circle before, I recommend taking a friend as it can be a powerful experience. My auntie visited Avebury (which is home to the largest megalithic stone circle in the world) and can't return because she was so overcome with a sensation that her skin was burning. We joke in our family it was because she was once burnt as a witch there, but it's also possible that she is sensing the energy of the stones. Many visitors have reported similar experiences.

Planting and harvesting: This is where Green and Hedge Witches thrive, but we can all create a herb garden in a window box, or care for potted plants. I have among my house plants at home: ivy, jasmine, poinsettias, a fig tree and a sweet little jade plant (to bring growth, renewal, and prosperity into my home).

Herbalism: Again, the realm of the Green Witch, using plants for medicinal and healing purposes.

Eco-living and environmentalism: Getting active in your role as earth guardian, working with kindness towards the earth.

Spells with Soil

Gardening is a stress reducer and mood lifter. The fact that there is now science behind it can add evidence to what many of us already instinctively know. *Mycobacterium vaccae* is a microbe found in soil that may encourage serotonin production, which makes you more relaxed and happier. Studies that were conducted on cancer patients found those who were exposed to it reported a better quality of life and less stress.

To work directly with the earth can be a very primal activity, in amongst dirt and bone, grass and stone. Such spell work is ancient, when witches worked with what they had, which was little, save what they could forage from Mother Earth. And while not for everyone, there can be a joy in getting your hands dirty in a real, down-to-Mother-Earth practical way.

☽ Dirt from an ancestral home or homeland may be used to help connect with the spirits of your ancestors or strengthen your connection to the past. You can also incorporate the dirt with that of your own garden to bring that ancestral connection home with you.

☽ Dirt from your garden can be used as an ingredient when you want to protect your home or the people in it.

☽ Get into the garden. The Kitchen Witch, Green Witch and Hedge Witch know the importance and value of plants and herbs for spells and recipes. The act of gardening itself is its own special magic.

Earth Elementals

Elementals are magical beings related to each element. They are personifications of an element or force of nature often mentioned in folklore, witchcraft and alchemy. Elementals (or earth spirits) live among plants and animals, looking after the natural world. They may well be part of the magic we feel when we are outdoors in nature, by oceans, rivers, amongst trees and mountains. Well-known earth elementals include fairies that, according to folklore, inhabit ancient ancestor sites such as stone circles and barrows. There is also the humble gnome who tends the earth through the seasons as well as cleaning

Earth Ritual

Plant a seed and tend it with love. If you are new to growing things, try nasturtiums. Sow the seeds into flowerpots or direct into the garden. These flowers are quick-growing and colourful enough to honour a goddess. And the Kitchen Witches among you may already know that their zesty, peppery leaves and flowers can be sprinkled onto summer salads and sandwiches. Nasturtium flowers represent vitality (probably helped by the fact that the plant is packed with vitamin C.)

Growing plants helps remind us that we cannot force ourselves into growth and transformation. Just like plants, things cannot be rushed. All we can do is give ourselves (and our plants) time, love and nourishment to find our own path to bloom.

the land of negative energy and pollutants (a big job!) Elemental beings are related to Mother Earth, so encounters with one, especially in Celtic traditions, are auspicious.

For every culture there are different archetypes of fairies. In Celtic lore, the fairy queens are also goddesses: Rhiannon and Áine, are both beautiful fairy queens and powerful goddesses. In English and Cornish myth, piskies, pixies, brownies and sprites live in trees and dance amongst flowers. In Icelandic culture the 'Hidden Folk' must be consulted before any new roads are built, to be sure of not disturbing fairy lands and incurring bad luck.

You may want to tune into elemental energies when working with the earth via witchcraft or yoga. Not only for connection with the planet but also connection with playfulness and whimsy. When you head outdoors to practice yoga or witchcraft tread carefully as you make your path upon the earth: there may be magical beings near! Perhaps ask permission as you walk into the woods. Take some time to listen in meditation to the symphony of earth elementals in the form of chirping birds, rustling leaves and seed pods dropping to the earth.

I am very aware of that look people can give you when you start talking about hidden folk and pixies. And that's okay, it is up to us how much magic and belief in such things we bring into our lives. Perhaps connecting to pixies and sprites helps you connect to your inner child and embrace fun in spells, rituals, witchcraft and yoga.

As I will say throughout this book, magic is where and how you find it. This journey of finding magic is not always a place for real and unreal: it is a place for intuition, feeling, joy and hope. Sometimes we may feel that we must be very serious in our spiritual practice (and sometimes this may be the case). But also, just because you're having fun, doesn't mean what you are doing isn't important, only that you are bringing joy to the process. So, giggle in yoga class, make a joke, allow yourself to laugh if you drop your crystals, or mix up your herbs, or forget the names of the goddesses. It's all okay! The care we put into rituals and practices is essential, it is mindfulness in action, but don't forget to embrace joy and fun as well!

Plant Magic

Just like us, plants and trees have their own energy – a vibrational frequency that is unique to each species. When we work with plant energy, we are connecting to the energy of nature, returning to ancestral knowledge and immersing ourselves within the blessings of the earth.

Fragrant oils and aromatic plants have been used for thousands of years throughout the world to transform consciousness, expand states of mind, connect to the divine, healing the body, mind and soul. They are interwoven with the history of yoga and witchcraft.

Attars – the most ancient form of essential oil process where the essence of the plant is 'held' in sacred sandalwood oil – are mentioned in ancient ayurvedic and yogic texts and, like yoga itself, originated from the Indus valley. Essential oils are our more contemporary Western version. Distilled directly from plant matter, essential oils speak to our senses, connecting to our innate healing powers – these healing gifts of plants and aromas are the spirit of a plant. Plants are multiskilled in terms of the healing qualities they can carry, composed of many that come together to form a whole. The Green Witch and Herbalist will likely know already that one plant can be applied to a multitude of uses, not just physical healing. We can approach plants from emotional and spiritual perspectives too. The more time you spend with one plant, the more of its transformational qualities are revealed.

Magic and transformation happens on a physical and emotional level when we allow the signature of the plant, expressed through essential oils, to become part of us. They can be our allies in deep soul searching and spiritual work. Perhaps a certain smell reminds you of your childhood home or homeland. If you wish to explore your ancestors and history, explore the herbs your grandmother and great-grandmother may have used. Maybe a grounding oil helps you cast your circle, or find calm during the high energy of the full moon.

Essential oils are also a form of herbal magic potion called a 'simple' which involves just one herb/plant (we learned about these in Chapter 7.) You may ingest a simple – such as a mint tea, whereas the majority of essential oils are for aroma only. You can use essential oils in so many ways: in a bath, in a diffuser, on a tissue, as a steam, in a base oil for massage...

The Power of Scent

As our first sense to evolve, smell is so powerful. All of our other senses are filtered through the thalamus, the part of the brain that processes what we attend to. Because we can't attend to every incoming message from our senses, it would be overwhelming. But smell goes directly into the limbic system. The limbic system is connected to our emotional life and memory, which is why smell and memory are so closely linked, and why smell is so emotive.

Oils that have the smallest molecules, such as mint, are known as 'top notes': they are the first we can smell and the first to disappear. We can also associate them with the higher chakras. In contrast a 'base note' is a heavier scent with bigger molecules, like cedarwood. We relate base notes to grounding and the root chakra.

Here are just a few ideas, using essential oils that are readily available. Always look for pure, organic oils that are sustainably produced. Remember that essential oils are sacred – carrying the soul of the plant and the wisdom of the earth – so use them with intention and respect.

Patchouli: This warm, soothing, and peace-inducing oil has been used for many centuries. Pharaoh Tutankhamun was buried with patchouli essential oil inside his tomb, and in Hindu myth, the Goddess Lakshmi favoured patchouli oil for embracing sensual abundance.

Cedarwood: Great for work with the root chakra or connecting to the earth element. Oils derived from trees all have grounding and stabilising properties. This oil can be used during times of stress to help focus the mind and steady the soul.

Jasmine: Jasmine oil has been used for centuries in parts of Asia as a remedy for anxiety and stress. The high vibrational energy of jasmine makes it perfect for supporting work in astral projection and meditation with the crown chakra.

Lavender: Lavender's properties include purification and the promotion of peace. You can use lavender to work into releasing tension, tightness and old hurt to create space to grow and transform.

Lemon: Lemon oil contains powerful antioxidants and boosts energy levels. Connected to the element of sun and fire, lemon is perfect for working with solar festivals, sun goddesses and manifesting.

Earth Magic for Yogis

In our practice, we can focus on our physical connection to the earth. But the earth is not just outside us: the earth element is represented in everything solid within the body: our bones, tissues and flesh.

I have found a variety of Earth Salutation variations over the years. But the version I use most often in my teaching is one I was inspired to create myself. It's a very simple version, that moves forward and backwards with the breath. *Bhumi* is the Sanskrit word for earth, as in soil, rather than the planet as a whole. You can see this sequence in action at **sentiayoga.com/yogaforwitches**

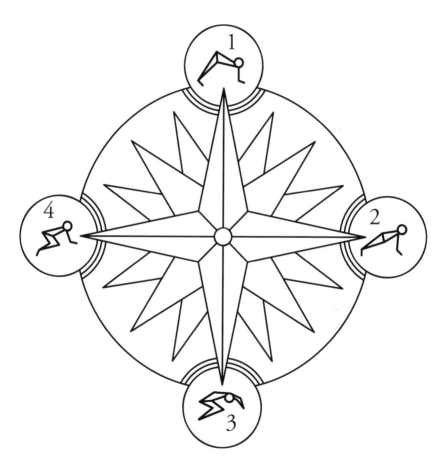

Earth Salutation Sequence

1. Downward Facing Dog – take an exhale here.

2. Inhale to move to High Plank.

3. Exhale to move to Child's Pose.

4. Inhale to move to Table Top position.

5. Return to Downward Facing Dog.

Cycle through easefully with the breath, 5 to 10 times.

Earth Goddesses

Most earth deities are female, representing the idea that the earth is the mother to us all.

Gaia (Greek) A personification of the earth and one of the primordial deities of ancient Greece. According to the creation myth of ancient Greece, primordial deities were the first goddesses and gods born from the void of chaos. The mother of all the gods, Gaia is also the home upon which they exist.

Cailleach (Celtic) The crone goddess and queen of winter. During the darkest months she sweeps her cloak of winter white over the land, freezing the ground. The personification of the elemental power of nature, the Cailleach is the creatrix of the land: she carves rocks and mountains to serve as her stepping stones.

Pachamama (Incan) Pachamama is a fertility goddess, mother of both earth and time. She provides everything needed to sustain life, presiding over planting and harvesting. She also embodies the mountains and earthquakes. One myth tells if you do not treat the earth with respect, Pachamama becomes a dragon beneath the mountains, causing earthquakes – a vivid reminder to honour her.

Aranyani (Hindu) Goddess of forests and the animals that dwell within them. Aranyani is freedom-loving, elusive, brave, and perfectly content in her own company, much like the many animals of the forest. There is a hymn in the *Rig Veda* (an ancient Hindu text) dedicated to her, which tells of Aranyani's love of her jungle home, even the dark corners, of which she has no fear. She's a wanderer and can easily hide from view in her lush green home but if you are lucky, you may hear her by the tinkling of bells on her anklets.

Prithvi (Hindu) Goddess of earth, her fertility is the source of all plants and nourishment of all living creatures. The Sanskrit word for the earth is *prithvi* and goddess Prithvi is the personification of the Earth Mother, the essence of the earth element. At funerals, prayers are said to Prithvi, that she may wrap the dead tenderly in her arms.

Papahanaumoku (Hawaiian) Usually referred to as Papa, Papahanaumoku is the Earth Mother and creatrix, who along with Wakea – Sky Father – created all people in Hawaiian lore. '*Hale o Papa*' – Papa's house – are temples in Hawaii for women to honour and worship Papa, her primordial power called upon to give life and to heal. Papa's spirit is that of the life-giving, loving, forgiving earth who nurtures all life.

Closing Thoughts

Let your roots connect you to your land and your ancestors. Working with and on the earth is a chance to realign and reconnect with the elements of the planet. And perhaps, most importantly, a chance to cultivate gratitude for the earth and its abundance: food, shelter and the very air we breathe are all precious gifts.

RITUAL AND CELEBRATION

The Sanskrit *r'tu* means sacred, both a special or sacred time or season, and specifically menstruation time for women (woman and rituals have always been intertwined!). A good thousand years later came the Latin word *ritus*, and eventually our modern-day word, ritual, which still refers to a special and sacred time.

Ritual uses symbolic actions and icons as a bridge between the physical and the divine. Rituals are often symbolic in their representation of a desired outcomes (i.e. a fruitful harvest) blessings on endeavours (i.e. a successful voyage) or an acknowledgment of a specific time of year. Ritual is a cultivation and embodiment of belief, respect and hopefulness as a group or as an individual practice.

Humans have used rituals since the dawn of conscious awareness to note the passage of time, celebrate special events, honour our ancestors, and seek advice from spirits. No matter your spiritual or religious background, rituals are a powerful way to stay connected with yourself and the earth. Magic is within all of us, but sometimes we lose touch with its presence and fail to see the incredible manifestations of energy in the world around us. Ritual can help us reconnect and listen.

Ritual can bring magic into the simplest of moments: lighting a candle, running a bath, brewing a cup of tea... The world is full of loud and large voices telling us so many versions of the tale of what we 'need' in life. Use your rituals to find peace – to reflect on what *you* need, and what you are grateful for.

Rituals can be an expression of our gratitude and bring us into synchronicity with our lives. The best rituals are unique and personal, so it's a good idea to explore and see what resonates with you. If you love to create, perhaps paintings or collages could play a central role in your rituals. If you are a singer, you could use your voice to chant and sing. You can and should use your own unique gifts so that you can create beautiful rituals that are personal, and that mean something to you.

Some of the most beautiful rituals can be made up on the spot. For example, last year, I went on a beautiful goddess retreat in Cornwall. And one of my favourite memories was standing on a clifftop by Tintagel Castle singing to the sound of the ocean in my own impromptu ritual.

Your rituals may be on your own or with others. Time spent with Mother Earth might include: lighting a bonfire, dancing, or creating a mandala from natural materials (like flowers, feathers, leaves, and stones). You may send prayers or light candles for a specific goddess, theme or element. Or enjoy spending time in nature with no fixed plan, just being with your friends or reflecting on your own, connecting to the earth. Rituals aim to calm and focus your active mind so that you can hear the quieter sounds of your intuition and magic. Solitary rituals such as meditation, self-care and relaxation may be done inside or out in nature.

Rituals can help you find peace, happiness and contentment within yourself; after all, your magic is part of you. But in a noisy world, it can be harder to tune into the wisdom we already know, which is how and why ritual can help. So the next time you come to a bridge, you may imagine you are stepping over a threshold, leaving behind any doubts and fears. When you are cleaning your home, you may imagine that as you sweep away dust, you are cleaning away self-judgment or criticism. Sweep away the old to create space for your fresh new sanctuary and good habits. This is how we weave ritual into our daily lives.

Making an Altar

A simple place to start with rituals or daily inspiration is to create an altar. This is a sacred space personal to you. A spot to display different goddesses, burn incense, and lay out candles and items from nature such as flowers, fruits, and feathers. You may use your altar as space to meditate, pray, or craft spells. You can change the images and objects with the seasons or as you feel inspired.

Creating an altar can call positive energy into your heart and home. It is a physical symbol of your intention, an invitation to that which you wish to invite into your life.

Select space in your home, one that you will regularly see, to remind you to take time to meditate or reflect. Make your choosing and cleansing of the area a ceremony in itself. You are acknowledging that you have chosen this space with intention.

Choose items that you feel connected to, such as elements or specific goddesses. My altar holds a goddess statue, images of the goddesses of earth and water, an amethyst crystal, a little bottle of water from St Nectan's Glen, feathers and candles. Your altar should be made up of items that you feel a connection to (rather than items you think you 'should' have). Feel free to get creative and play with arrangements. There is no right or wrong way. Some mornings I light a candle and meditate, stretch and write by my altar. Other days I create an evening ritual or spell. At Yule time each year, my Christmas tree becomes my altar, and I love to practise yoga, meditate and journal beside its light.

Many witches like to have a symbol of the four earthly elements on their altar. For example, a feather or incense for air, crystal or stone for earth, a little bottle of water or seashell for water and a candle for fire. Different coloured candles may be used for different spells. You may also wish to use a bowl or cauldron, an athame (ritual knife), a totem or witch bottle (see below), a wand, a ritual cup or chalice for your rituals. And finally, your Book of Shadows, which you may keep on your altar at all times or only bring it to the altar when you wish to craft a spell or ritual.

Witch Bottles

Witch bottles are bottles filled with various objects and liquids as a form of protection. More recently, they have also been used for healing, prosperity and abundance. The witch bottle is essentially a bottled spell – a form of witchcraft that dates back hundreds of years. Witch bottles have been found buried under the fireplace, under floors, and plastered inside walls of ancient dwellings. You can fill a witch bottle with anything you wish, depending on your intentions.

The Yogi Witch Bottle

This witch bottle is one I have created especially for your yoga witch journey!

☾ *Find a (preferably glass) bottle or small jar with a good lid. Make sure it is clean.*

☾ *Write a positive affirmation or sankalpa (intention) on a small piece of paper. What is it you are seeking on your journey? Strength? Freedom? Joy? Inspiration? Write it down and roll or fold it up to go into your bottle.*

☾ *Add some herbs and spices native to Asia, yoga's homeland:*

  ○ *A few black peppercorns for protection on your journey, and an acknowledgement of the most ancient uses of a witch bottle: as protection from negative or evil energy.*

  ○ *A star anise, used to bring good luck, love, and health.*

  ○ *A small stick of cinnamon for protection, strength and success.*

  ○ *A few dried petals from a blue lotus, sacred to Hindus and revered by yogis. The thousand-petaled lotus represents spiritual illumination, wisdom and knowledge. The lotus flower grows in muddy waters, rising above the surface to bloom like the enlightened being who emerges from the noise of the world. (You can buy dried blue lotus flower petals from herbal shops like Neal's Yard and online. You could also use lovely little lavender flowers – which are purple in colour, like the crown chakra and also represent purity and spirituality).*

☾ *A ribbon to go around the bottle neck: violet or blue for the crown chakra (or you may choose a colour of one of the other chakras that resonates with you).*

☾ *Something of yourself to claim it as yours – some hair, a fingernail clipping or something from your home.*

☾ *Once you have prepared and sealed your bottle, place it upon your altar or a sacred space, or you may wish to bury it in yoor front garden or a window box to bring protection and enlightenment to all who dwell within.*

Morning Ritual

You can also begin to combine some of the yoga witch practices that we have learned so far in this book into your daily routine to create a morning ritual.

☽ Start by stirring up some energy/prana/chi: stretch, move, do a few rounds of Sun, Earth or Moon Salutations (look to Moon, Sun and Earth Magic Chapters) depending on your mood/energy levels. We are just starting to connect body, breath and mind.

☽ Sit in a comfortable position and focus on your breath as you allow yourself to settle and ground in a simple meditation to bring your mind to focus (Refer back to Chapter 4 for meditation ideas). Open up the space for self-reflection and self-expression without judgment or expectation.

☽ Start writing: You can be intuitive with your writing, it could be freestyle or you might start with a word or phrase that resonates with you (you can refer back to the journal prompts in Chapter 6). Or you may simply create a list of goals for your day.

☽ When you come to a natural stop in your writing, pause, and return to your meditation. Observe any thoughts and feelings that have arisen, you may want to write them down too. When you feel ready, close your journal and move into your day.

Let us start with one of the most basic acts of ritual that can be made wherever you are, whatever the occasion: casting a circle.

Casting a Circle

When taking your first steps into the world of pagan and witchy practices, and indeed many nature-based beliefs, you are going to come across a *lot* of significant circles, wheels and spirals. After all, we are talking about connecting to a great circle: our earth. In the sky, the moon and sun are two more special circles. So, in a way, it's no wonder that you'll find wheels outlining the seasons, elements, directions, moon phases, cycles of death and rebirth, the cycle of life, without beginning or end.

The most common use of circles in witchcraft is 'casting a circle', which means to draw a circle around yourself during spells as form of focus and/or protection. It may be a physical circle or created in the mind's eye. Once a circle is cast, one may or may not then call in the directions. The Wheel of the Year and 'calling in' are ways of orienting oneself, both physically on the land with the calling in of directions and one's place in time cycles.

How to Cast a Circle

Casting a circle can help focus your attention and energy for a spell, ritual or grounding. And it is, literally, a circle around you or your group. The circle can be physical, such as a ring of candles, leaves, salt... They can be used to form a complete circle or placed at North, South, East and West – using the items to symbolise the directions just like on your altar. You can also imagine a circle around you. At the beginning of a spell or ritual, you create the circle, either physically or in your mind. You can, if you wish, also call in the directions at this point.

At the end of your ritual you then 'open the circle', physically and/ or mentally. You may want to thank the directions/elements, i.e. "Fire, you were here, and I thank you". A lovely and common closing, especially when working in a group is: "The circle is open, but never broken. Merry meet, and merry part and merry meet again."

The Four Directions

For those unfamiliar with 'calling in' the directions, of East, South, West and North, this is a grounding and orientation exercise: literally acknowledging the directions around you. The four directions are deeply embedded with symbolism. Each direction has key associations, sometimes known as elementals or correspondence, that are all connected: North and winter can occupy the same space on some wheels, as can South, summer and the element of fire. There are varying ideas about which element, direction and season are laid out around the Wheel so you may find Wheels that have the water element associated with summer, air with winter, and fire with spring. And different layouts for southern and northern hemispheres of the earth. You are, of course, welcome to create a Wheel that feels right to you!

Calling In the Directions

If you are new to calling in the directions, an example of what this might look like can be helpful. But please remember this is just a guide. I have been learning about how to call in the directions as part of my priestess training at the Glastonbury Goddess Temple. It can feel a little odd saying it out loud at first, but now I find it a lovely addition to many of my meditation classes and rituals. I also find it useful when leading classes on retreats abroad – to orientate oneself in a new land and honour our arrival. One of my biggest hurdles when learning to call in the directions was getting what I thought was the 'script' right, when in fact all is needed is the intention behind the words. So don't worry too much about the exact words, and keep them as simple as you wish: let intuition guide you.

Upon opening a ceremony, you may want to say something like "Greetings", "Bright Blessings" or "Hail and welcome!" and on closing something like "Thank you and farewell". When calling in the directions, most often we start with East, spring and the rising sun.

EAST/SPRING/AIR/EQUINOX

I call in the energy of the East. Place of the rising sun, new beginnings and ideas, air and winds, the place of enlightenment and illumination, new day and new dawn. The East that represents spring.
Hail and welcome, energy of the East!

SOUTH/SUMMER/FIRE/SOLSTICE

I call in the energy of the South. The power of summer and abundance. Place of the noonday sun, place of passion, creation and inspiration. The spark of life, the fire within.
Hail and welcome, energy of the South!

WEST/AUTUMN/WATER/EQUINOX

I call in the energy of the West. Place of the setting sun, of reflection and introspection, place of endings and transition. The power of autumn's bountiful harvest, evening dreams, place of transformation and change.
Hail and Welcome, energy of the West!

NORTH/WINTER/EARTH/SOLSTICE

I call in the energy of the North. Of night and winter, the place of peace, rejuvenation and stillness, inner wisdom, and reflection. North star and new moon.
Hail and welcome, energy of the North!

Seasonal Celebrations

In traditions around the world, rituals and celebrations welcome in and mark changes in the yearly cycle of the sun, outlining fundamental activities of survival such as planting and harvesting. These changes were celebrated. Each new season brought change and our ancestors found value in each. There is a harmony to working with these seasonal energies that we have lost in modern life: our culture tends to enforce one way of being as superior.

Seasons, the change and connection from one type of energy to another in the world, are key to both yogic and witchy wisdom. Seasonal celebrations help us to connect the movements of sun, moon, earth and ourselves into a cosmic dance, understanding that there is flow and a cyclical nature to these changes. The rituals of yoga and witchcraft celebrate and make space for the different seasons of being by celebrating the changing seasons outside, helping us to grow in wisdom by making connections with the changing energies within each of us. Rituals encourage us to celebrate each, and support us in traversing the in-between times, as we learn how to transition from one to the other.

Not only can reconnecting to these seasonal celebrations help guide us in our own connection with each season, they can inspire us to create or take part in larger ritual celebrations each year.

Wheel of the Year

The Wheel of the Year is a way of looking at life in a circular rather than linear manner. The circle and spiral are ancient feminine symbols. Masculine energy is more often portrayed as a straight line.

The Wheel of the Year is divided into eight and follows growth through the year: plant a seed at Imbolc, it grows through spring equinox and ripens over summer to be harvested at Lammas, Mabon and Samhain. The ground lays dormant over Yule to be re-awoken once again at Imbolc. You can use this circular thinking for the cycle of the moon as well, and you could have a circle representing a lunar month. Some goals you have may take a year to work through, some you may do in a month. While the Wheel of the Year/Medicine Wheel/Wheel of Life varies by culture, it honours the belief that all things on earth have an energy force, and all things are interconnected.

So let's look in more detail at the festivals that track the journey of the sun's position in our skies as we journey round it though the year. And outline the seasons within the framework of the Wheel of the Year. Then we can explore how you might connect to and enjoy these seasonal changes on a more personal level.

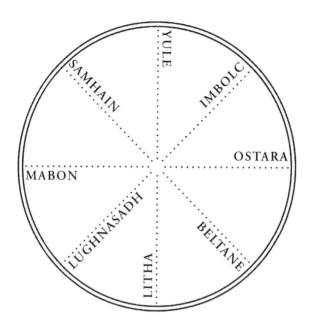

Equinox and Solstices: The Solar Festivals

Solstice means when the sun 'stands still'. Winter and summer solstice are times to celebrate and honour the returning or departing of the lighter days. You'll see as we look at the sabbats that summer solstice is also known as Litha and winter solstice as Yule.

Equinox meaning 'equal nights' is when day and night, light and dark are poised in perfect balance. Spring equinox is also called Ostara and autumn equinox is often referred to as Mabon.

In-between the solar festivals are the cross-quarter, fire or sabbat days of Imbolc, Beltane, Lughnasadh/Lammas and Samhain. These festivals represent the cycle of birth, life, death and rebirth. Be aware that many modern Wheels of the Year, including this one I've outlined below, have been pieced together from various elements of Celtic, Gaelic, Pagan and Anglo-Saxon cultures and so you may well see variants on this theme.

The Sabbats

Winter Solstice or Yule
Northern Hemisphere: Dec. 21/22
Southern Hemisphere: June 21/22

The shortest day. From this day forth, the days grow longer. Its name is derived from Middle English *yol* and Old English *geōl*. This pagan midwinter festival signals the gradual returning to the light.

Imbolc
Northern Hemisphere: Feb. 1/2
Southern Hemisphere: July 31/August 1

Imbolc is a Celtic word, meaning 'in the belly or womb', and the festival is dedicated to fertility. Imbolc celebrates the first stirrings of spring and the first sparks of new life.

Spring Equinox or Ostara
Northern Hemisphere: March 21/22
Southern Hemisphere: September 21/22

Named after the Germanic goddess of the spring and the dawn: Ostara/Eostre. Ostara brings new beginnings, fertility, rebirth and renewal. The natural world is coming alive, the sun is growing in strength, and the days become longer and warmer. Those sparks at Imbolc are transforming into abundant fertility at Ostara

Beltane
Northern Hemisphere: April 30/May 1
Southern Hemisphere: Oct 31/Nov 1

Beltane means 'bright fires ' or fires of Bel, the Celtic god of the sun. This celebration is an honouring of life at the end of spring and the beginning of summer, when earth energies and life are at their peak.

Summer Solstice or Litha
Northern Hemisphere: June 21/22
Southern Hemisphere: Dec 21/22

The Anglo-Saxon name for June and July is Litha, so the name is often used for midsummer festivities. Midsummer is the longest day of the year, and brings abundance, joy and warmth.

Lughnasadh/Lammas
Northern Hemisphere: Jul. 31/August 1
Southern Hemisphere: Feb 1/2

Lughnasadh is one of the four ancient Gaelic seasonal festivals, along with Samhain, Imbolc and Beltane. It is named after Irish sun god Lugh. Whereas the English/Anglo Saxon word for this festival is Lammas (meaning loaf/bread). It marks the beginning of the harvest season, a time for gathering in and giving thanks for abundance.

Autumn Equinox or Mabon
Northern Hemisphere: September 21/22
Southern Hemisphere: March 21/22

Named after the Welsh god, Mabon, son of the earth goddess, Modron. At equinox, night and day are again of equal length and in perfect balance. But from now on the year begins to wane and from this moment the nights become longer than the days. This is the second harvest when we gather in the sweet fruit harvest: apples, pears, and berries.

Samhain
Northern Hemisphere: Oct. 31/Nov 1
Southern Hemisphere April 30th/May 1

Of the various ideas about the root of this word, my favourite origin story is from the Celtic word *samani* that means assembly or coming together, but it also translates as 'summer's end'.

At Samhain, the darker half of the year commences. This fire festival is a particularly magical time for many pagans, as it is their beginning of the new year. With the commencement of this dark phase comes the invitation to rest and reflect on the past year, and to envisage new beginnings. Samhain is the last harvest festival of the year. As the last of the nuts and berries are gathered in, we reach the end of this yearly cycle of birth and growth.

Working the Seasonal Energies

The time in between each festival also has its own unique energy and significance, which can be honoured and acknowledged in ritual, spellwork and yoga practice. I've suggested practices to nurture your creative spirit during each of the seasons. Your inner yogi, witch and creatrix may just need a little encouragement to emerge or this can be a reminder to reconnect. After all, the witch, yogi and creatrix energies live within us all, just as the changing energies of the seasons do.

Stirring: Imbolc to Spring Equinox

Reawakening: Spring Equinox to Beltane

Growing: Beltane to Summer Solstice

Thriving: Summer Solstice to Lughnasadh

Gathering: Lughnasadh to Autumn Equinox

Harvesting: Autumn Equinox to Samhain

Surrendering: Samhain to Winter Solstice

Resting: Winter Solstice to Imbolc

Stirring (Imbolc to Spring Equinox)

Stir with your inner yogi: With movement explorations – self-enquiry, nurture and nourishment.

Stir with your inner witch: Plant both seeds and intentions ahead of Ostara and spring equinox. Connect to nature, deepening your awareness of your natural surroundings.

The sap is rising again, think about intentions as you prepare to cross the threshold into a new burst of life in this year.

Stir with your inner creatrix: Create a sacred space in honour of this season: it may be an altar, a meditation space, or a cleansing of your home.

Reawakening
(Spring Equinox to Beltane)

Reawaken with your inner yogi: Focus on building energy and vitality: think Sun Salutations and Vinyasa yoga. And play with movement outside in nature – acro-yoga in the park perhaps!

Reawaken with your inner witch: Focus on reconnection to the earth – grounding, nurturing and healing from the inside out. Connect with nature and develop your presence.

Reawaken with your inner creatrix: Think about working with thresholds as you enter spring: you can hang a witch bottle by your door for prosperity or plant roses to invite love into your home. You can work with thresholds with meditation and visualisation as you step into a new season.

Growing (Beltane to Summer Solstice)

Grow with your inner yogi: Explore drive and motivation, but also intuition – as you work towards challenging poses you want to 'master' make conscious decisions in your movements.

Grow with your inner witch: Seek your own healing medicine through movement and nature's offerings. There is so much that can nourish us: forest bathing and a little time in the sun can help us bloom.

Grow with your inner creatrix: Connect to your primal spirit: move, dance, play in nature. Listen deeply to rhythms and inspiration that arise.

Thriving (Summer Solstice to Lughnasadh)

Thrive with your inner yogi: Connect to your inner fire and power – move with intention and confidence as you embrace your version of each pose. Think strong warriors and perfectly imperfect balances! Explore your edges, but be empowered not to push into pain. Moving out of your comfort zone is great – but don't rush the process!

Thrive with your inner witch: Time to explore your relationships with yourself, others and nature. Explore boundaries, honesty and self-honouring.

Thrive with your inner creatrix: Express gratitude, joy, abundance in your favourite creative forms: paint, dance, journal, bake and craft!

Gathering
(Lughnasadh to Autumn Equinox)

Gather with your inner yogi: Explore fluid movement – being in flow with body and breath. Gather in a feeling of gratitude for the abundance of wonder that is your beautiful body.

Gather with your inner witch: Gather herbs, flowers, wood and seeds in the late summer sun to add to your altar or spell supplies.

Gather with your inner creatrix: Explore and celebrate ways to get closer to nature while the weather is still warm: organise a beach clean, a tree planting, or track animal footprints.

Harvesting
(Autumn Equinox to Samhain)

Harvest with your inner yogi: Practice gratitude, non-judgement and non-criticism in your yoga practice.

Harvest with your inner witch: Reflect under the September full moon, known as the Harvest Moon. Consider what you've worked for: where has your path led you? What fruit has grown from your actions?

Harvest with your inner creatrix: Create beautiful and nourishing foods with the harvest of nature: jams, soups and wine will bring joy and sustenance!

Surrendering
(Samhain to Winter Solstice)

Surrender with your inner yogi: Explore ways to release safely through movement. Practice letting go and embrace the art of surrender and rest.

Surrender with your inner witch: A time for cutting ties and finding ways to release all that no longer serves you. Take some time to face your shadows and heal.

Surrender with your inner creatrix: As we are slowing things down, coming back to the ground, you may wish to explore your stories and ancestral heritage.

Resting (Yule to Imbolc)

Rest with your inner yogi: This is a time for silence and stillness: think yin yoga and meditation.

Rest with your inner witch: Enjoy this chance to rest and explore your dream time. Why not record your dreams or journey as the Hedge Witch through meditation and visualisation.

Rest with your inner creatrix: Create light in these darkest months: make candles, bright altars and bring your own sources of light and joy to the darker evenings.

Goddesses of Seasonal Celebration

The goddess archetypes each bear their own gifts and guidance for us; we merely need to welcome them to speak, lead, and inspire us from day to day. Rituals and other intentional practices can bring us into the present moment, helping us to open our minds to receive wisdom from our guides and reconnect us to our magic.

Ostara (Anglo-Saxon, Germanic) The goddess Ostara, or Eostre, goddess of spring, the east, rebirth, and the dawn. She is usually depicted as a maiden, and beautiful like the spring season itself. Ostara is the name of both the spring goddess and the spring festival in March. This is a time to celebrate the rebirth of the land, fertility, abundance, and welcoming back light and life after the dark winter. The sun is returning, and with it comes hope and warmth.

Ostara represents spring's life force and earth's renewal, and it's a good time to think about renewal in your own life. At the time of Ostara, you may want to decorate your altar with symbols of the season. Think about all the colours you see in nature during spring: bright daffodils, crocuses, tulips, green shoots – you can bring them onto your altar. Spring is a time of fertility and life, so the egg is the perfect representation of the season, as well as symbols of animals such as baby rabbits, lambs, and chicks.

Persephone (Greek) is a dual goddess who reflects the separation of the seasons: light and dark, and transitions of spring/summer and autumn/winter. Hades, god of the underworld, fed Persephone a single pomegranate seed – having tasted food from the underworld, Persephone was committed to staying there. But via the diplomacy of her mother, Demeter, an arrangement was made that Persephone could return to the earth each spring. Just like a seed, Persephone spends the dark months of the year below the surface, and when she returns to the earth's surface, light returns. The earth rejoices in warmth and abundance, and Persephone is full of gratitude when she gets to rise in spring. It is always useful to visualise the year as a circle or wheel, to remind us that no matter how dark the day, however lost we may feel in our own 'underworld', spring will return and we will get to turn once more to face the sun!

Closing Thoughts

Celebrate! Celebrate each new day, month, season and lunar cycle. Find the rhythms and cycles in the year that help you find connection. Create your rituals to celebrate and honour these moments. Your daily rituals do not need to be complicated or even planned – but take time to enjoy little moments of wonder as they arise! Your days do not always have to be perfect, but let them mean something to you: something learnt, something released, something honoured… Ceremony and ritual can be a time to carry yourself and your soul in a sacred way. But it's not the only time to do that. Rituals remind us that we are sacred, and teach us how to carry ourselves in a sacred way every single day.

SPREADING
THE MAGIC

B oth witchcraft and yoga may be solitary practices that heal and sustain us as individuals. But when shared, they become more powerful. They also have the possibility of helping impact our actions on the world.

By practising together, coming together – whether that be in yoga, magic or any craft – we raise positive energy together: we rise together. We support each other in taking the right action – in being kind to ourselves, to others, and to the planet. In this way we can spread magic through ourselves, others, the planet and beyond. Spread love, and you'll spread magic. Throw it around like confetti! Because a world filled with magic is special, indeed, even for those who refuse to see it. In whatever way you let magic in your life, enjoy it, claim it, live your magic. Share and spread magic with love!

Women's Circles

The most powerful classes I teach are groups of women. Groups of women that feel safe enough in a space held in love to laugh, to cry, and to talk. I teach school teachers, dog trainers, healers, counsellors, jewellers, writers…some so rarely get the chance just to be, and to take some time to listen to their hearts. To let out emotions if they want to, to talk if they want to. For those without a coven, the yoga room or meditation space can be a place to feel that magic: the magic that happens when women come together…and create. This is what we do best. We create a welcoming space, a space to be heard, a circle. So, more than anything, through this chapter I implore you to find a tribe, circle, coven, a group who lift you up and who listen with love to whatever it is you need to say. To be held in a space of love with others is a support we all need at some point.

Something that has always happened in groups I have held space for, is that as soon as people start sharing, they realise that they are not alone, that everyone has very similar doubts, fears and challenges. To hold a loving, accepting space can also help us let go of pressure to get it 'right' or feeling a sense of comparison or competition with the person next to us. When we feel safe, we can let go of some of that fear that we somehow need to prove ourselves, or give the impression that we are working hard. We can accept what all of us already know (*smarana* again!): we are all doing the best we can. There is a real relief in letting go of having to prove that in any way. To feel safe with other people has such a huge impact on wellbeing and mental health. Connection with others (in a way that is right for us) is essential for a meaningful and happy life.

Loving Kindness Meditation

This meditation is called *metta bhavana*, or Loving Kindness. It comes from the Buddhist tradition and is a practice in cultivating love. I think it's pretty special; I hope you do too. You may well recognise this meditation from yoga and meditation classes you have already taken. This is a version I have tweaked over the years, but you'll find a similar outline to all metta meditations.

Metta bhavana is a technique of developing compassion. We begin with sending love inwards, to ourselves, for unless we love and accept ourselves, it's difficult to extend love to others. As we open to deeper levels of compassion, we journey towards breaking though blocks that we may feel toward ourselves or toward others.

Take a comfortable position in a space where you can feel relaxed and comfortable. Allow your breaths to be calm and restful as you begin to settle into your peaceful space. Breathe in and breathe out with ease. In your mind's eye, imagine yourself in a place of nature. It may be a garden, a beach, a meadow overlooking an ocean. It may be somewhere from your memory or imagination; it is somewhere you feel safe and calm. Allow yourself to take in your surroundings – perhaps the sun on your face, or a scent of flowers.

As you settle and relax here you realise that there are four other people here with you in this place.

The first person is someone you will be able to bring to mind easily because this person is you. Take a moment to visualise standing in front of your own self. Visualise your face, hair and clothes.

And here you say, in your mind's eye:

May I be happy,
May I be loved,
May I be safe,
May I live with ease.

And to your own heart, you send a beam of light and love.

The second person is someone you love and feel positively about. It may be a family member or partner. Take a moment to visualise their face, maybe imagine the clothes they are wearing and the colour of their hair. And to this person, in your mind's eye, you say:

May you be happy,
May you be loved,
May you be safe,
May you live with ease.

And from your heart to theirs you send a beam of light and love.

Then we move onto the next person. This is someone you feel neutral about. It may be someone who served you in a cafe or someone who you work with. You have no strong feelings for this person. Take a moment to visualise their face, maybe imagine the clothes they are wearing and the colour of their hair. And to this person, in your mind's eye, you say:

May you be happy,
May you be loved,
May you be safe,
May you live with ease.

And from your heart to theirs you send a beam of light and love.

Now, the final person is someone you feel negatively about. It may be someone who has hurt you in the past or angered you. And even though you may not want to, take a moment to visualise their face, maybe imagine the clothes they are wearing and the colour of their hair. And to this person, in your mind's eye, you say:

May you be happy,
May you be loved,
May you be safe,
May you live with ease.

And from your heart to theirs you send a beam of light and love.

And the beams of light that shine out to these four people now shine out past them, past your space and out into the world, circling the entire globe, and reaching you once again, like the sun shining upon your back.

May all beings be happy,
May all beings be loved,
May all beings be safe,
May all beings live with ease.

Allow yourself to bask in this light for a few minutes.

Goddesses of Love

Kuan Yin (Chinese) Goddess Kuan Yin is known as the Goddess of Mercy, and her speciality is compassion. One of my favourite Kuan Yin myths is that in her first life, she was born as a man who sought to help guide souls on their journey to enlightenment. Overwhelmed with an endless cycle of lost souls, he despaired and shattered into a thousand pieces. From his remains, the gods shaped him as a woman, a goddess: more suitable for compassion and mercy in unlimited quantities. In some depictions, she has a thousand arms and eyes in each palm, so that she can see our distress and reach out to encircle us with love. According to another myth, when Kuan Yin was about to enter heaven, as she stood on the threshold, she heard the cries of humanity. She did not enter but returned to help all who suffer on earth. When you send out a mantra, chant or spell, maybe it's Kuan Yin who hears you...

Kuan Yin is associated with the colour white, with precious stones such as pearls, rose quartz, pink tourmaline, jade and emeralds. In the plant world she is symbolised with lotus blossoms and willow branches.

Freyja (Norse) may well be the most renowned of the Norse goddesses: a lady, a queen, a witch and a goddess of love. In charge of love, fertility, and death, Freyja rules over the land of Folkvangr as Queen, and there she receives the souls of half of those that die in battle (the other half go to Odin's hall in Valhalla).

Freyja, which translates as 'lady', had many roles in the ancient Norse belief system. She was skilled in *seidr* – a Norse term for sorcery relating to the telling and shaping of the future. Freyja is credited with teaching witchcraft to other gods and humans.

Closing Thoughts

Love and gratitude: two of my favourite words. And so well intertwined. To love our body, we must be grateful for it, as it allows us to journey, dance and practice yoga. Cherish with gratitude the specialness that it is to find love. In whatever form it takes. We never know for how long we will have it. So I implore you, express gratitude and appreciation to those you cherish, to things you cherish, luxuriate in activities you love. Because there will be a day when they are no longer available to you. So love now, for now is all we have.

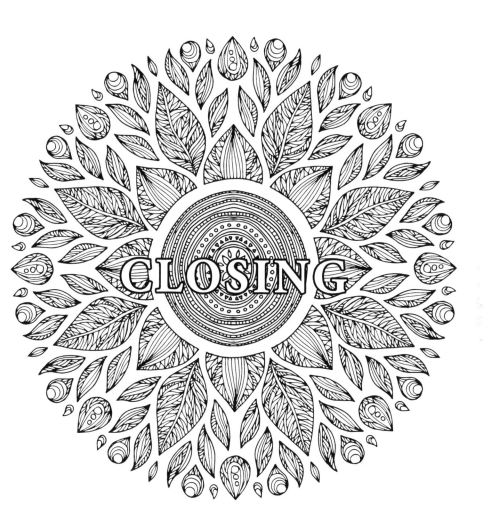

W hen I come to the end of each yoga class, I often say, "We'll end this practice as we started..." which usually involves reconnecting to the breath.

So, in this journey, let's end this as we started: the pursuit of magic.

Together we've explored some ideas and inspirations in two realms of spirituality and magic that are special to me; I have utterly relished the opportunity to share some of this journey with you. Yoga and witchcraft are two of many gateways into deeper levels of being and of connection. The witch and the yogi walk in a balance of earth and energy. They connect to ancient knowledge of healers, guides and teachers. Witchcraft and yoga are both lifelong paths of self-education. A celebration of the interconnectedness of all things from the fascia of our body to the seasons of the year.

I hope this book has given you some ideas about finding your own magic and answered some questions you had...as well as posing some new questions that you might want to explore further.

Fiction is so fantastic because it transports you to another world, and it may well stay with you long after the story is over. But with books like this, the end of the book is really just the beginning. Now...well, now you have work to do!

Go forth and use this book as fuel and inspiration. Use the exercises within as ideas to follow and inspire. Share it with others. Something very special happens when groups of magical people get together: whether that group be yogis, witches, crafters… Reach out and find your circle, your tribe, reconnect with old friends, and support your sisters. These connections will help you find the magic within, and open your mind and imagination to what can be created.

With such vibrant visual and physical practices such as yoga and witchcraft, there was too much glorious imagery to fit into this book, so alongside the book, you will also find a website which can be your resource. As well as a Facebook group where we can gather together and continue our journey beyond these pages. It doesn't end with this book. There is so much more to find and discover!

Yoga and witchcraft are forms of empowerment for taking control of your life, body, mind and heart. They are powerful tools that can help you to take steps towards creating your own life. This magic is about so much more than we can see. Magic can work in mysterious ways – it can turn up as a person, a teacher, a loved one, a new friend, an opportunity, a new job or adventure.

Magic is a path you can walk, through magic, you can open to ecstatic experience and freedom. Magic invites you to treasure who you are and treasure all of life upon the earth. We can choose to honour life in all its mystery. We can decide to treat each other with kindness and celebrate our marvellous differences while still united as residents of Mother Earth.

I believe that a woman empowered can be such a force of nature as to create wonder in the world we may call magic. Many of us have become disconnected in some way. Separated from ourselves and what we are capable of. Because of this disconnection, the simple act of listening intuitively to our bodies can be something so amazing as to be called witchcraft... and maybe it is, it's certainly special.

To quote a section of my Wake the Witches Meditation (see the full script in Appendices)

It is a reminder that there is the power of magic within us all. Over the years, we have been separated from our power, our intuition, our knowledge of the natural world and its rhythms. But here, my beautiful witches, as we once again take hold of our cape and wrap it around us, we begin to remember...

We begin to connect, to align with magic that runs through us all.

And as you walk through nature by moonlight, you may find yourself picking a sprig of mint to cool and calm, chamomile to soothe, or maybe a rosebud for love. And I am sure that you already knew what these flowers and plants mean – without me even saying. Because deep within your blood and bones there is knowledge. Knowledge of the women that came before you. Knowledge of the healers, the herbalists, the wise woman. These are the witches. They are not cruel or evil. They are healers. They are helpers. They are creators. This is the legacy of the wise woman. The legacy of connection with the natural world that runs within all our bones, our blood and our hearts. And as you take your quiet walk through the woods, each of the women on this journey feels this connection to each other and to the world. As we take this journey to reclaim what is already ours: a knowledge, and intuition and a connection that has always been within us.

We are reconnecting to the elements, reconnecting to our intuition and reclaiming the knowledge of our ancestors. Reclaiming the power that was always within us. Here, in this place, beautiful sisters, we reclaim the witch, we reclaim our inner wise woman. We reclaim the woman who knows. The woman who sees. The woman who is power.

Don't ever let someone tell you how to find your magic: they don't know, they can't know who you are and appreciate the magic that runs through your veins. It may be that you believe and relate to everything you have read in this book. Perhaps not.

The vital question – woman, witch, goddess – is, *do you believe in yourself?*

Namaste, witches!

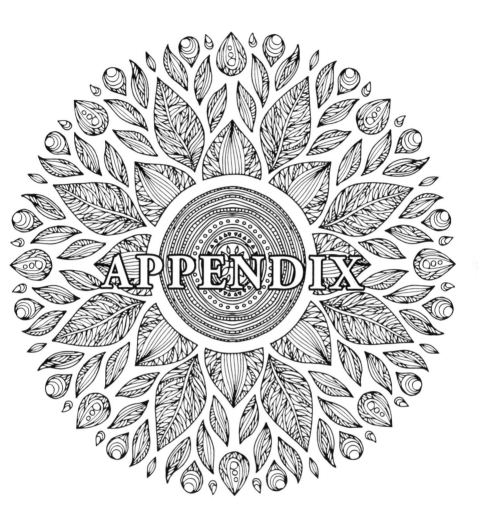

Meditation Scripts

I adore leading meditations. When I was a child practising yoga, meditation was my favourite time, and one of the first CDs I ever bought was ocean sounds to meditate to. It was with these soothing tones playing that I took my first steps aged seven into meditation and the simplest of spells and incantations. (These were not sophisticated attempts – they would usually involve mixing creams together to make beauty potions!)

I draw my themes for meditation from the seasons, the lunar calendar and the goddesses. Sometimes I'll also use oracle cards, pulling some during the meditation and using their message as my guide for the group.

You can use these scripts as a guide for your own meditation. You may wish to record yourself reading through the script, or read them at group meditations. Or read through as a story to inspire reflection, artwork or journaling. I attempted to pick meditations that relate to some earlier chapters: the moon, goddesses, and chakras, but these are also just some of my favourites! And I'll finish with two very special meditations I created especially for this book "Wake the Witches" and "*Yoga for Witches* Oracle Messages Meditation".

If you enjoy listening to meditations, I can wholeheartedly recommend the app Insight Timer. It's free and features thousands of beautiful meditations, including my own; which you can find under *Sarah Robinson – Sentia Yoga*.

Moon Magic Meditation

If you can, do this under a full moon, it's all the more special. But you can connect to full moon energy anytime you wish.

Allow yourself to relax, close your eyes, feel comfortable and supported by whatever is beneath you: cushions, mat or blanket. And take some time here as you settle the body into comfort. Allow the breath to be calm and unhurried. We'll take our time to reconnect to calm and peace before we begin to work our moon magic…

Allow each inhale to draw in a sense of peace and restfulness, and every exhale a release of anything you would like to let go of.

So, you can inhale peace and exhale fear; inhale calm, exhale anxiety… Allowing each and every inhale to draw in that which comforts and nourishes you, and each exhale to let go of anything that no longer serves your highest good.

And right now, whatever season and time of day, and whatever stage the moon is at above you, we are going to visualise a beautiful large full moon above us in the sky. The moon is our constant companion here on earth, and she is so closely linked with goddess mythology. She represents the feminine, the cycles, the ebbs and flows of bodily rhythms and earthly rhythms. Goddesses Selene, Artemis, Diana and Hina are all there, within the moon's sacred energy.

And here, in our place of rest, moonbeams stream down from the full moon, bathing us in silvery light. Imagine these bright beams of light washing away whatever tensions and tightness you have gathered, washing away busy thoughts of deadlines and shopping lists. This bright full moon light is cleansing and comforting, nourishing like a warm hug.

In your mind's eye, envisage yourself moving into a beautiful open space. There is grass beneath your feet as you gaze towards the moon. Here we can more clearly see the full moon above us. We find ourselves barefoot standing on the soft green grass, each blade gently illuminated by the moon's soft light. We walk, with no sense of hurry, across this green space. We come across a band of beautiful women, each holding a lantern in her hands, like a constellation of earthly stars. The light of the lanterns illuminates the women's faces. They smile at you, kind and welcoming, and you have a sense that they have been expecting you. They turn and begin to walk away, and you know that you must follow. Walking in peace alongside these beautiful beings, you feel quietly excited that great things may be afoot.

The trail of lanterns leads you through a wooded glade, the glowing light of the moon shines down upon each and every one of you in this peaceful procession. As you come to a clearing amongst the trees, the women with their lanterns create a great circle around you. One of the women steps forward. In her arms she holds the most beautiful gown of silver, greys and whites, sparkling in the moonlight. You put on this gown, it feels so soft and warm, almost as though the material has been infused with love and light.

You stand here in the moonlight surrounded by this ring of lanterns, this ring of stars, this ring of beautiful women, maybe you see them as women you know, or perhaps they represent each of the lovely moon goddesses around the world. Maybe you see them as wood fairies and flower sprites. Whatever friendly force feels comforting to you.

As you step into the middle of the circle, a huge felled tree has left a giant circular table for you, on which to work. And on top of this tree trunk is everything you need to create your own special moon magic tonight. There are bowls and little sparkling glass vials of liquid. There are candles of every colour of the rainbow. There are incense and herbs and flower petals. A beautiful apothecary of everything you could dream of. It all looks exciting, unusual, and yet familiar.

You start by taking hold of a bowl. It is smooth and warm to your touch. It might be made of wood, or clay, or metal or glass – visualise the colour and material of this beautiful bowl you hold within your hands. And as you gaze into this bowl, you know instinctively what it is you wish to manifest on this beautiful night. You know which kind of magic you want to invoke: bravery, or healing, or joy, or love, or peace. Take your time to conjure this word in your mind, allow yourself to visualise it fully in your mind's eye.

And as you look at all the little bottles and bowls in front of you, you know exactly which ones to use to create your magic moon potion tonight. Pick the petals, herbs, oils, tinctures and extracts that you need. Allow your mind to gather all the beautiful items and mix them together in your bowl of manifestation on this beautiful moon night.

Perhaps you take a handful of rose petals from one bowl to represent love, perhaps shiny pearls from another to represent strength, maybe beautiful coloured oils for joy. You may choose perfumes to represent sensuality and white feathers for harmony. Allow yourself to gather as many items to pop into your bowl as you wish. Take your

Yoga for Witches

time to envisage them and what they mean to you.

You stir all these beautiful items together in your bowl with a bright silver spoon, and as all these things come together, they make the most beautiful coloured liquid within your bowl. It shimmers like the night sky, with purples and pinks and blacks all swirled together like a galaxy, little dots of sparkle shine brightly within the liquid. And once again you bring your mind to what you wish to manifest this night.

You hold the word in your mind, but to the group of lantern bearers around you, it is as though you have said it aloud. They have heard you.

And you raise your potion to the sky, each and every one of the lanterns around you is also raised high. Allow the moon to bear witness to your hopes, your dreams and your manifestations.

As if the moon has heard you, it grows just a little brighter, shining a stronger light into your circle, shining such bright light onto your lantern bearers that they burst into light and disappear.

And with your bowl, you know what to do: you gently pour the liquid all over your body like a warm shower of light as you cover yourself for a moment in this liquid, this potion, this mixture of galactic colours. The liquid is so warm and beautifully scented. Bask for a moment, covered in colour, covered in magic, covered in moonlight. Almost as soon as the liquid has coated you, it sinks into your skin and disappears – you are clean and dry once more, still wearing your beautiful lunar robes.

And as the time comes to leave this circle of light, now empty of lantern bearers but still beautifully lit by the moon above, you can continue to wear your robes, comforting you as you place down your bowl on the tree trunk, ready for the next time when you wander into the woods to celebrate the full moon.

White Light Chakra Meditation

Get into a comfortable position, sitting or lying down. Feel your breath moving in and out of you as you relax. Feel your body softening into the surface beneath you. Allow your eyes to softly close.

Take your attention to the space just above the top of your head where your crown chakra abides. Imagine that above you there is a pure white lotus bud, glowing with light and energy.

Envisage this glowing white lotus bud rotating slowly as the petals unfurl until they are open wide and flat. Light and warmth shine upon your crown chakra from this special flower, and you feel the light warming and soothing the top of your head.

This light moves down through your third eye chakra and throat chakras, filling these wheels, and you, with light. Light and warmth are growing as you feel this light filling your body, charging each cell with love.

The light moves through the heart chakra, the solar plexus, sacral and finally, the root chakra.

Your entire body is filled with light. It is so full, that the light within you shines out, creating an aura of white; a shield that can protect you from the slings and arrows of life, protecting your energy.

Continue breathing in the radiant light energy, getting a sense now that every cell in your body has been charged and filled with light. Bask in this light for a few quiet minutes, feeling how it is both nurturing and reviving – like a warm hug.

Taking a couple of deep breaths, become aware of your physical body now. Begin to wriggle your fingers and toes. Feel yourself coming fully back into your physical body and maybe take a stretch. You may place your hands to rest on your heart or any chakra. Relax and allow the energies of love and light to continue to sparkle within every cell of your body.

Wake the Witches Meditation

Before you settle down for our meditation to reclaim our inner witch, I want you to find some material: a blanket, a throw, a dressing gown, a towel that you can wrap around yourself. This will help you feel cosy and comfortable. But more than that, my darling, today this material you wrap around yourself is going to represent your witches cloak.

This is a cloak of our innate power as women and witches. It is a reminder that there is the power of magic within us all. Over the years, we have been separated from our power, our intuition, our knowledge of the natural world and its rhythms. But here, my beautiful witch, as we once again take hold of our cape and wrap it around us, we begin to remember...

We begin to connect, to align with magic that runs through us all.

And as you settle and relax in your comfortable place, allow this blanket of warmth around you to represent anything you need in this moment. It might be love, healing, forgiveness, strength...

Allow yourself to be wrapped in this feeling and feel yourself begin to relax. As the eyes gently close and the breath begins to calm, we find ourselves settling into peace...into restfulness...

As we allow the body to settle into stillness and into calm, we find ourselves in our mind's eye, standing barefoot on soft green grass. Above us, the night sky shines with moonlight and starlight. And as we envisage this space, we see the cloak that we are wearing is transformed... It may be transformed with colours, sparkles or sequins. It may be decorated intricately with leaves, animals or symbols. Allow yourself time to visualise yourself standing tall, your feet grounded on the earth, beautiful cape wrapped around your shoulders.

You feel connected and calm in your surroundings. Each of the elements is here. Your feet rest on the earth and the gentle evening air swirls around you. The warmth and fire of the stars above you and also your inner warmth and inner fire. And the water of the blood running through your veins. Each element is here with you. And you connect to this space.

Around you, tall trees reach skywards. And as you stand, taking in your environment, you see, slowly, more women, walking barefoot in the grass, each with her own cloak of magic and beauty. The women emerge from the trees and you join them on a slow and easeful walk to a special place. As you walk on the earth you feel the connection with the ground, you pass under low branches of leaves and fruits and blossom, and you thank the trees for the shelter they offer you as you wind into the woods.

And as you walk through nature by moonlight, you may find yourself picking a sprig of mint to cool and calm, chamomile to soothe, or maybe a rosebud for love. I am sure that you already knew what these flowers and plants mean – without me even saying. Because deep within your blood and bones there is knowledge. Knowledge of the women that came before you. Knowledge of the healers, the herbalists, the wise woman. These are the witches. They are not cruel or evil. They are healers. They are helpers. They are creators. This is the legacy of the wise woman. The legacy of connection with the natural world that runs within all our bones, our blood and our hearts. And as you take your quiet walk through the woods, each of the women on this journey feels this connection to each other and the world. As we take this journey to reclaim what is already ours: a knowledge, and intuition and a connection that has always been within us.

We arrive in a forest clearing. The trees encircle you keeping you safe and sheltered. Above you, the night sky shines with moon and stars. And your group of women create a circle, holding hands, a kaleidoscope of colours and faces and souls come together in this circle.

Feet on the earth, sending heart skyward. Connecting in circle. Connecting in sisterhood. Reconnecting to the elements, reconnecting to our intuition. And reclaiming the knowledge of our ancestors. Reclaiming the power that was always within us. Here, in this place, beautiful sisters, we reclaim the witch, we reclaim our inner wise woman. We reclaim the woman who knows. The woman who sees. The woman who is power.

And as you and this group of women gaze to the sky, a flash of light – a shooting star – crosses the sky. You feel empowered by your time with the witches, your time with the ancestors, your time with your sisters.

Finally, you release the circle, releasing each others' hands. And as you part on this great moon night, you know you can reconnect and reclaim whenever you wish. The circle is open but never broken.

You can stay here in your power, in your safe place, for as long as you wish.

Blessed be, my witches.

Yoga for Witches Oracle Messages Meditation

When I got to the end of this section, I thought back to the intro- duction, where I mentioned drawing oracle cards to inspire the meditation, and I thought, "Well, I better do a special one for all the awesome folks reading this book!"

So, under a full moon in January I pulled four cards from my favour- ite goddess deck to guide me. I asked the deck if there was a message I should pass on to the readers of this book. During the recording, I pulled the cards and just spoke what came to mind as they turned. And I have transcribed the meditation here! Created especially for this book, and you, dear reader! (I was a little nervous about this draw in case, well, I'm not sure, what if the message wasn't what I wanted for the book? What if I didn't know what to say about the cards? And I was determined to do it just once. As it turned out, as it always turns out, I think the message from the oracle and goddesses are perfect! As is always the way with oracles, this message may mean something to you now, or maybe something that is of use in the future.)

Welcome, woman, witch, goddess!

This is your time, so take as long as you need to find a soft, warm, comfortable space to be. A place where you can feel supported and set down the weight you carry upon your shoulders. A place where you can fully surrender and be supported in the hands of Mother Earth beneath you.

Allow your breaths to be easeful, slow and unhurried, each deep inhale drawing in anything you wish to draw in, and each deep easeful exhale letting go of anything you wish to let go of as we take a journey to meet the goddesses and what messages there may be for us today.

Allow yourself to sink into a restful place of peace and calm, a place of intuition, of compassion and kindness. A place of magic and spirit and of listening to our own heart, our own breath, and our own inner voice.

And as we leave the busyness and the comings and goings of the outside world behind us for a short time, we'll envisage that we are resting in a place in the natural world. Somewhere where we can see the night sky. We may find ourselves in a garden or park, on a beach or on a cliff beside an ocean. We may find ourselves in a wooded forest or an open meadow. You may visualise yourself anywhere from memory or imagination. This beautiful place of nature can be anything you need.

Allow your senses to absorb the imagined space around you. What can you see? Are there tall trees surrounding you? Can you smell flowers and plants on the night air, or is it the salty scent of seaweed and ocean mists? Is it the deep citrus scent of pine needles or jasmine floating on the warm night breezes? Can you feel the surface beneath you? Is it soft green grass or warm crumbling sand?

Allow yourself to fully visualise this special place, your special place.

And as you gaze to the skies from this place, you see a beautiful shining moon above you and sparkling stars creating sparkles of light on a velvety sky. Deep, dark and warm, the night sky surrounds you like a warm blanket.

And from your place of taking in your surroundings, you see for the first time a beautiful flickering bonfire. Dancing and casting shadows through the evening air. And around this bonfire are four figures, each wearing beautifully coloured robes that sparkle and glint in the firelight. You feel drawn to join them in the circle. And as you complete this circle around the fire, there are now five.

You and these four very special beings have been drawn here to-night. Like the five elements of earth, air, fire, water and ether. Five have come together this night to convey and hear a special message.

In unison, all five of you take a seat around the fire and wordlessly. As they take down the hoods of their robes, you see their beautiful faces for the first time. Before you are four of the goddesses, four very special beings, and it may be that you see these four aspects of the divine feminine as women that you know and love, you may see them as light or sparkle, you may see them as colours or energy. They may not fully form in your mind until we are introduced to each one… but already as these four faces look at you with such kindness and compassion, you know that the messages that they have for you will be delivered with love and sage counsel.

The first beautiful goddess to address you is the Roman goddess of wisdom, Minerva. Here, in this aspect, she represents beliefs. And her wise words for you are these:

"Carry your chosen beliefs carefully. The time has come to discard beliefs that no longer serve you, that weigh you down, that hold you back. It is time to invest belief in yourself, your own power, your own beauty and your own skills."

You thank Minerva for her message and her love and take a moment to absorb what she has said to you.

The second goddess is the divine feminine archetype, the Lady of Beasts, the Sumerian fertility figure. She is often seen surrounded by animals, who connect to her cycles of fertility, of looking after her young, of guarding carefully those she loves. And the Lady of Beasts is here today in this circle to bring you a message on relationships. Her message is this: "As you begin your important journey. Seek out and claim who you are."

The Lady of Beast is the creatrix, and just as she creates, she encourages you to create relationships and groups of support that nurture and nourish your highest good. Take a moment to reflect upon what she has told you and thank her for her message and her love.

Our third beautiful goddess is the Hindu goddess Lakshmi, the goddess of abundance. Her message for you is to celebrate abundance in all its forms and nurture abundance in your life. To celebrate your skills, your powers. "You are abundance. You are limitless!"

Take a few moments to absorb the messages that Lakshmi has

passed onto you here and thank her for her love.

And our final goddess to turn to you in this circle is the Japanese goddess of the sun, Amaterasu, the goddess of beauty and sunlight. Here in this form, she brings you messages to encourage you and gently guide you towards power, freedom and the illumination that awaits you on your path. "You are beautiful!"

As you absorb these words from Amaterasu, you feel the warmth and light of the fire, the warmth and light of the goddesses shine upon you, and you bask in the light and wisdom they have passed on to you today.

And with a smile, you know it is time for the goddesses to leave as the glow past the horizon signals the coming of the sun, the coming of power. Light and illumination is on its way. And as the sun peeks over the horizon, the first rays of light cast golden shadows and all at once, the goddesses are alight with warmth and glow, and they are gone.

You are left here with your thoughts and the comfort and love that they have brought to you today. And you feel that amongst their words is a little wisdom that means something special to you that you can take with you on your journey, knowing that they will watch over you as you take your steps, as you learn and grow. Embracing the power within, the power that is always within you, the power you possess as woman, witch and goddess.

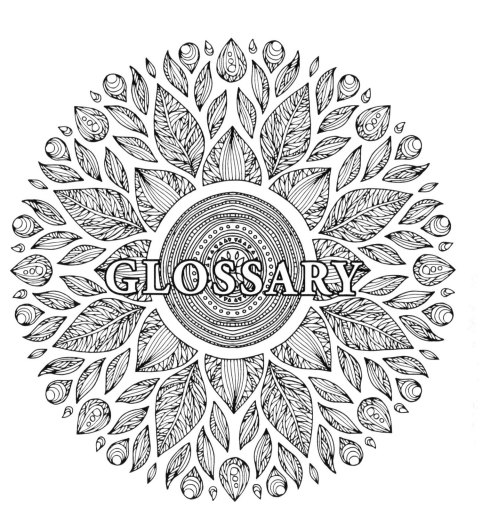

GLOSSARY

Witches

Witch

The wise one. One who practices magic, which may or may not include practicing spells, charms, rituals and ceremonies. Various etymological roots include the Old English words *wicca* and *wicche* meaning wise. And *weik* meaning to bend and wind.

There are of course, as many kinds of witches as there are people, and you can call yourself whatever you wish. Some of these names were new to me but so gorgeous I had to include them! Moreover, it also helps show you can be literally any kind of witch you like. You can specialise in any area; you may directly call yourself a witch or may want your title to reflect your area of passion/expertise.

Crystal Witch

Witches who work with crystals and precious stones, such as crystal healing, crystal meditation or chakra balancing. A Crystal Witch has extensive knowledge of stones, including how to identify them and to use their properties.

Eclectic Witch

This witch picks and chooses from many traditions to create her own form of witchcraft to meet her own needs and abilities. This style is similar to Chaos Magic.

Faerie Witch

Has a focus on the Fae (goblins, elves, fairies, sprites), mythology, and their relation to the natural world.

Green Witch

A witch whose practice focuses on nature, natural materials and energies. Green Witches are often skilled herbalists, gardeners and wildcrafters. Green Witches attune to the cycles of nature and see all natural places as sacred.

Hedge Witch

A Hedge Witch is a witch who has knowledge and skills about herbs and also astral projection and divination. She and acts as an intermediary between the spirit or astral realms and the material realm.

Kitchen Witch

A Kitchen Witch or Hearth Witch focuses their magical practice on the home and hearth. Kitchen Witchery often involves the use of essential oils, herbs, foods and everyday objects.

Sea Witch

The Sea Witch is in tune with the energies of the sea and feels a close and physical connection to the rhythms and power of the sea.

Yoga Witch

I'm certainly not the first to blend these two elements together. Look up #YogaWitch on Instagram and you'll find over twenty-five thousand images! But I am honoured to have done my part to cultivate the idea of the Yoga Witch: one who weaves wisdom, practice, and holds space for others on their yoga journey.

The Various Branches of Witchcraft

Paganism

An umbrella term covering a wide range of beliefs. It can be applied to many non-mainstream religions. In different circles, the word pagan is used to describe any earth-based spirituality.

Chaos Magic

This school of magic emerged during the late twentieth century in England. Popular techniques include creating sigils. Sometimes referred to as "success magic" or "results-based magic", chaos magic emphasises the attainment of specific results.

Dianic Wicca
A recent tradition of Wicca. Originating in the US in the 1970s, this is a feminist tradition that focuses on the sovereignty of the Goddess.

Druidry
Druidry is a spiritual movement that promotes harmony, connection, and reverence for the natural world.

Folk Magic
A set of magical practices and beliefs common to a particular community or culture. Folk magic is practical, intended to bring about a real, physical change, such as soothing burns and calming headaches.

Wicca/Gardnerian Wicca
This is a modern/neo-pagan religion that was introduced to the public in the 1950s by Gerald Gardner. Wiccans are taught witchcraft as part of their spiritual experience. There are many Wiccan traditions, specific beliefs and practices differ between covens. Wiccan moral and value system is summed up by The Wiccan Rede.

Witchy Words

Altar
A space used as the focus for ritual, especially for making offerings to a deity and working with spells.

Athame
An athame (pronounced: *ath-uh-may*) is a blade used in ritual and spellwork. In Wicca, the athame is (usually) black handled and its purpose is strictly symbolic.

Book of Shadows/Grimoire
A written record of spells, magic and magical correspondence. A Book of Shadows can be handed down through generations and used to record anything a witch desires or deems appropriate. Some covens and Wiccan groups have stricter rules about one's Book of Shadows.

Calling In
Calling In is a ritual performed at the start of magical or spiritual work. It is a summons to elemental energies tied to the four directions of the compass into a magic circle.

Casting a Circle
During spellwork and rituals, a circle is cast to define the sacred ritual or workspace. This circle is a construct of energy, its purpose can vary by tradition.

Cauldron
The cauldron is a symbol of transformation and rebirth. Cauldrons can represent the female aspect of divinity, the womb, and are used in conjunction with wands, swords and athames to reflect the divine feminine and masculine.

Chalice
The chalice is used in rituals in a variety of traditions, sometimes to hold liquid. It can represent the female element and the element of water.

Correspondence
Charts of symbolic connections in the natural and magical world. Tables of correspondence help us connect and group together elements for spell and ritual work. For example, the moon corresponds to colours of silver and white. You can use existing correspondence from books or work to create your own.

Coven

A coven is usually a small community of witches and/or Wiccans who regularly gather for special occasions. Covens may gather to share knowledge, honour Sabbats or Esbats and/or to work magic spells.

Elemental

Elemental spirits are associated with each of the four elements. The names of the elementals vary, but the most common are: Earth elementals – gnomes and pixies. Water elementals – nymphs and mermaids. Air elementals – sylphs and angels. Fire elementals – salamanders and dragons.

Equinox

When the sun crosses the celestial equator. When the hours of daylight and darkness are equal. There is an autumnal equinox and a spring equinox each year.

Esbat

Esbats are special days for covens to convene, or witches to dedicate for spellwork. They may take place on either the full or new moon, or both depending on tradition.

Manifestation

This is the writing down or focusing on what you want to bring into your life. One may perform a manifestation spell, ritual, meditation, or create manifestation bottles, boxes and bowls.

Power Animal

A power animal embodies the characteristics of the species it represents, as an archetype of that animal. Animals may appear as guides, aids and advisors for specific life phases. A power animal may also be referred to as a spirit animal, a spirit guardian, guide or a totem.

Sabbat

Holidays and feast days celebrated by pagans including Wiccans and traditional witches. Depending on the tradition, there are usually four or eight Sabbats in the year following the pattern of the Wheel of the Year. Some groups celebrate the four Celtic fire festivals as Sabbats. These are Imbolc, Beltane, Lughnasadh and Samhain. Others celebrate the equinoxes and solstices as Sabbats as well.

Scrying

Scrying is a divination method that involves looking into a reflective surface such as a scrying glass or a crystal ball. Witches gaze into the surface, or past it, to achieve a trance-like state, where visions may appear.

Sigils

A sigil is a picture that represents a desire or intention. They are most commonly created by writing out the intention, then condensing the letters down to form an icon.

Simple

A simple is a remedial potion using a single herb, used for healing.

Smudge

A smudge stick is a dried herb bundle that is burned and made to smoke to cleanse a space, a tradition that originates from many Native American traditions. Many yoga teachers have adopted this practice (me included). Burning a sage smudge stick, the fragrant wood palo santo or incense, which is more traditionally used in yoga traditions, helps to create a sacred space for yoga and meditation.

Solstice

Solstice is the two annual extremes of the sun's height in the sky. At summer solstice, the sun reaches its highest point of the year and we receive the longest day. At winter solstice, the sun appears lowest in the sky and we have our shortest day.

Spell

A spell is an intentional focusing of energy to achieve an objective. Spells are traditionally written or spoken, the power of words and intention being vital.

Wand

A wand is a stick (most often made of wood) used for ritual work. They are associated with masculine energy and air or fire elements depending on the tradition. Wands can be used for focusing energy, and for stirring.

Wiccan Rede

The Wiccan Rede is a poem, often summed up by its line "An ye harm none, do what ye will", created by Doreen Valiente in 1964. It is thought of as the basic ethical code of the various branches of Wicca that adhere to it. There are various versions of the Wiccan Rede, and interpretations may vary between covens. Non-Wiccans may subscribe to a similar idea, or not.

Witch Bottle

A witch bottle is a magical tool that has been in use for centuries, as a protective spell. Witch bottles once included sharp objects such as pins and bent nails to ward off evil.

Sanskrit words

Asana

Physical posture.

Ayurveda

The 'Science of Life', considered the sister science of yoga.

Chandra
Moon.

Dosha
In Ayurvedic philosophy, we embody the elements in different ways.
Our dosha refers to our specific 'type' of elemental qualities.

Mantra
A sound or chant, often used in meditation. A mantra can focus concentration on one purpose and can help still the mind.

Mudra
Hand position or seal for directing prana.

Namaste
A classic greeting and parting phrase for yogis and Hindus, with many translations around honouring to one another, my favourite is "The light in me honours the light in you".

Prana
Life force, vital energy. Known in Chinese cultures as *chi*.

Samsara
'Wandering' or 'world', with the connotation of cyclic change. It also refers to the cycle of death and rebirth.

Samskara
In yogic philosophy, samskaras are the mental imprints left by all thoughts, actions and intents that an individual has ever experienced: the subtle impressions of our past actions.

Samyama
Holding together, binding, integration. The combined simultaneous practice of *dharana* (concentration), *dhyana* (meditation) and *samadhi* (union).

Sankalpa
Intention.

Sanskrit
Ancient Indian language thought to have inherent power.

Seed mantra/bija
Specific one syllable sounds such as 'Om'. From these seeds great things can grow!

Siddhis
Attainment, fulfilment and/or power.

Smarana
'Remembering', 'uncovering'.

Surya
Sun.

Svadhyaya
Introspection and 'study of self'.

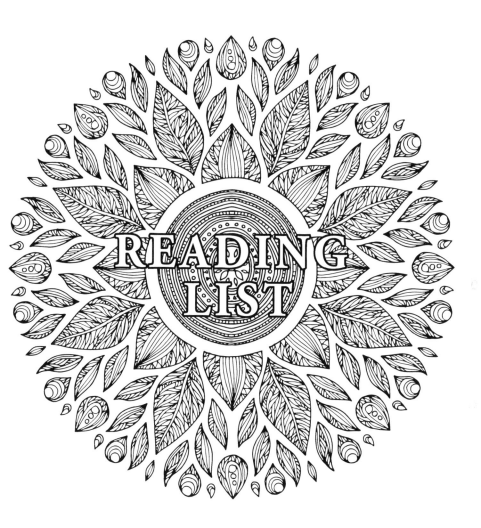

M y first ever yoga book was gifted to me by my first yoga teacher Tina because, aged 11, I wrote her a poem about yoga. That book was *The Beginner Bear's Book of Yoga* by Rosamund Richardson and James Ward. At the front, Tina wrote, "May you continue to enjoy your yoga". I still have this book, and I continue to heed Tina's precious words!

The following is in no way an exhaustive list, but a few books I have found invaluable in my continued study of yoga and magic! I haven't referenced many works in the book itself as I tried to navigate telling my own story. But all of these books helped inspire and inform my work, and I hope you find them useful too.

Yoga

Hatha Yoga Illustrated – Martha Kirk Brooke Boon and Daniel DiTuro
Yoga Sutras of Patanjali – Edwin F. Bryant
Art of Attention – Elena Brower and Erica Jago
Yoni Shakti – Uma Dinsmore-Tuli
The Spirit of Yoga – Cat de Rham and Michele Gill
Everyone Try Yoga – Victoria Woodhall
Eight Lectures on Yoga – Aleister Crowley. (Crowley is a controversial character for sure. In this book you'll find sections called 'Yoga for Yellow Bellies' and 'Yoga for Yahoos', it's a strange and fascinating read! And to suggest that yoga and magic are lovers is a wonderful analogy!)

Magic, Witches and Women in their Power

Green Magic – Robin Rose Bennett
The Witch in Every Woman – Laurie Cabot
Wheel of the Year: Living the Magical Life – Pauline Campanelli
The Book of English Magic – Philip Carr-Gomm and Richard Haygate
The Oxford Illustrated History of Witchcraft and Magic – Owen Davies
The Magical Year – Danu Forest
Witchcraft: A Very Short Introduction – Malcolm Gaskill
Witchcraft and Society in England and America, 1550-1750 – Marion Gibson

Waking the Witch – Pam Grossman
Witch – Lisa Lister
Burning Woman – Lucy H. Pearce
Medicine Woman – Lucy H. Pearce
Real Magic – Dean Radin
The Earth Path – Starhawk
The Spiral Dance – Starhawk
How to Turn Your Ex-boyfriend into a Toad
– Athena Starwoman and Deborah Gray
Weave the Liminal – Laura Tempest Zakroff

Goddesses

Warrior Goddess Training – Heatherash Amara
You are a Goddess – Sophie Bashford
Naming the Goddess – Trevor Greenfield
Goddesses – Sue Jennings
Priestess of Avalon, Priestess of the Goddess – Kathy Jones
The Goddess Oracle deck and book – Amy Sophia Marashinsky
Goddess Wisdom – Taniska
The Inner Goddess Revolution – Lyn Thurman
Goddess Rising – Lyn Thurman
Dancing in the Flames – Marion Woodman and Elinor Dickson

ACKNOWLEDGEMENTS

Many amazing women, witches and goddesses came together to help me on this journey.

A huge thank you to Lisa Nelson for her illustrative talents and creation of the yoga salutation diagrams, and to Adriana Hristova for the most magical cover.

Fellow Yoga Witches Trish, Tam and Kat for reading through my first drafts. All my dear friends for your enthusiasm and encouragement! And my Goddess Temple teachers Nikki McAuslan (Swann) and Marion Brigantia.

To Lucy H. Pearce, for being my inspiration and mentor, and for bringing me and my book into the Womancraft family.

And to my Dan for his love, support and kindness in the face of great weirdness and witchery!

ABOUT THE AUTHOR

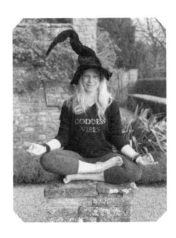

Sarah is a yoga and meditation teacher based in Bath, UK (once named after a goddess: the ancient Roman town of Aquae Sulis). Her background is in science; she holds an MSc in Psychology and Neuroscience and has studied at Bath, Exeter and Harvard Universities.

Sarah has practiced yoga since the age of seven. Weaving in her love of all things myth, magic and goddess, Sarah is passionate about creating magic to inspire and transform. Through yoga, meditation and ritual she aims to help everyone connect to their own special magic and inner power.

ABOUT THE ARTISTS

Cover Artist: Adriana Hristova

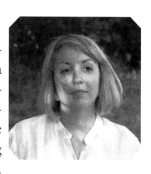

Adriana Hristova is a Bulgarian based freelance visual artist and illustrator. She has a Bachelor's degree in Fine Arts, a Master's degree in Printmaking and is currently working as a Visual Arts teacher. Her artworks are deeply inspired by nature and all its living creatures, paganism, mythology, folklore, naïve art and often carry a symbolic meaning or a universal message. Through her art, Adriana wishes to inspire love and appreciation for everything that surrounds us – the seen and unseen, the small and the large, the material and the spiritual.

Instagram @adrhristov

Internal images: Lisa R. Nelson

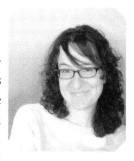

Lisa is an accomplished illustrator and painter. She lives in beautiful rural Massachusetts where she enjoys communing with nature while kayaking the Nashua River, biking on rail trails, or volunteering with shelter dogs. She would like to thank her wonderful and supportive boyfriend, Christopher Johnson, who patiently recreated all of her illustrations digitally for this project.

PainterLisa.com

ABOUT
WOMANCRAFT

Womancraft Publishing was founded on the revolutionary vision that women and words can change the world. We act as midwife to transformational women's words that have the power to challenge, inspire, heal and speak to the silenced aspects of ourselves.

We believe that:

☾   books are a fabulous way of transmitting powerful transformation,

☾   values should be juicy actions, lived out,

☾   ethical business is a key way to contribute to conscious change.

At the heart of our Womancraft philosophy is fairness and integrity. Creatives and women have always been underpaid. Not on our watch! We split royalties 50:50 with our authors. We work on a full circle model of giving and receiving: reaching backwards, supporting TreeSisters' reforestation projects, and forwards via Worldreader, providing books at no cost to education projects for girls and women.

We are proud that Womancraft is walking its talk and engaging so many women each year via our books and online. Join the revolution! Sign up to the mailing list at womancraftpublishing.com and find us on social media for exclusive offers:

(f)   womancraftpublishing

(y)   womancraftbooks

(o)   womancraft_publishing

Signed copies of all titles available from
shop.womancraftpublishing.com

YIN MAGIC

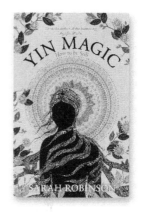

SARAH ROBINSON

Yin Magic shows how ancient Chinese Taoist alchemical practices can mingle with yoga and magic to enhance our wellbeing from sleep to stress-levels, helping us to move beyond burnout cycles and embody the beauty of letting go. It shares:

☾ What yin is…and why it matters.

☾ An introduction to the practice of yin yoga

☾ Yin yoga journeys for each season and the meridians.

☾ Insight from cutting-edge neuroscience research.

☾ Connections between Celtic, witch and Chinese medicine traditions.

☾ Sympathetic magic and how to bring it into your yoga practice.

☾ How to embrace the magic in the darker times of night, new moon and winter.

Yin Magic helps us to make everyday magic at a sumptuously slow pace as an antidote to the busyness of modern life.

KITCHEN WITCH

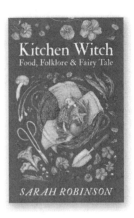

SARAH ROBINSON

Welcome to a place of great magic – the kitchen!

Magic, superstition, cooking, and food rituals have been intertwined since the beginning of humankind. *Kitchen Witch: Food, Folklore & Fairy Tale* is an exploration of the history and culture of food, folklore and magic and those skilled in healing and nourishing – herbalists, wise women, cooks, cunning folk and the name many of them would come to bear: witch.

Kitchen Witch is an invitation to see the magic in every corner of your kitchen. With the Kitchen Witch as our guide, we'll explore food, nature, magic, and transformation. We'll discover what the name of Kitchen Witch could mean to us in modern interpretations of ancient practices. May this book of stories and ideas show that there's magic in the mundane, witchcraft within your walls and the Goddess really is in the details.

Within this book you'll find no recipes, but something cooked up just for you; you'll find stories – stories of magic, healing, and hearth, of feasts and fasts and fairy tales. Of poisoned apples, bewitching gingerbread, and seeing the future in a teacup…

Wild & Wise: sacred feminine meditations for women's circles and personal awakening

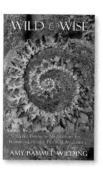

Amy Bammel Wilding

The stunning debut by Amy Bammel Wilding is not merely a collection of guided meditations, but a potent tool for personal and global transformation. The meditations beckon you to explore the powerful realm of symbolism and archetypes, inviting you to access your wild and wise inner knowing.

Suitable for reflective reading or to facilitate healing and empowerment for women who gather in red tents, moon lodges, women's circles and ceremonies.

> *This rich resource is an answer to "what can we do to go deeper?" that many in circles want to know.*
> **Jean Shinoda Bolen, MD**

Burning Woman

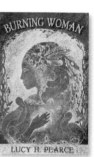

Lucy H. Pearce

A breath-taking and controversial woman's journey through history – personal and cultural – on a quest to find and free her own power.

Uncompromising and all-encompassing, Pearce uncovers the archetype of the Burning Women of days gone by – Joan of Arc and the witch trials, through to the way women are burned today in cyber bullying, acid attacks, shaming and burnout, fearlessly examining the roots of Feminine power – what it is, how it has been controlled, and why it needs to be unleashed on the world in our modern Burning Times.

> *A must-read for all women! A life-changing book that fills the reader with a burning passion and desire for change.*
> **Glennie Kindred, author of *Earth Wisdom***

Creatrix: she who makes

Lucy H. Pearce

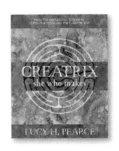

"Creatrix is a more accessible identity for us to claim, especially as women, than the archetype of Artist, which has been forged in the male image for so long.

"To live as a creatrix is to dedicate your life to nurturing and sharing your creative gifts, using them in every way you can to imbue the world with greater colour, beauty, joy, understanding, playfulness, daring, rebellion…"

From bestselling author of *The Rainbow Way* and *Burning Woman*, comes *Creatrix* – a soul-full companion for the road less-travelled, to support the life that unfolds when we say YES to The Creative Way.

This definitive guide covers vast territory, from owning our creative gifts and our voices, claiming space and time to create, the dynamics of the creative process, to the key parts of Creative Entrepreneurship from marketing to building soul-led communities.

Moon Time: living in flow with your cycle

Lucy H. Pearce

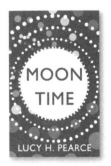

Hailed as 'life-changing' by women around the world, *Moon Time* shares a fully embodied understanding of the menstrual cycle. Full of practical insight, empowering resources, creative activities and passion, this book will put women back in touch with their body's wisdom.

This book is a wonderful journey of discovery. Lucy not only guides us through the wisdom inherent in our wombs, our cycles and our hearts, but also encourages us to share, express, celebrate and enjoy what it means to be female! A beautiful and inspiring book full of practical information and ideas.

Miranda Gray, author of *Red Moon* and *The Optimized Woman*

Dirty & Divine: a transformative journey through tarot

Alice B. Grist

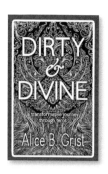

Wherever you are, whether beginner or seasoned tarot practitioner, *Dirty & Divine* accompanies you on a powerful personal intuitive journey to the depths of your existence, encompassing the spectrum of wisdom that the cards offer.

> *What I find REALLY juicy about this book, is that you'll experience how to use the cards + the stories, metaphors, signs + symbols they hold as a tool to help you remember your power. The fierce self-love, the courageous + wild truth of who you were before you forgot.*
> Lisa Lister, creatrix of www.thesassyshe.com, author of *Love Your Lady Landscape* and *Witch: Unleashed. Untamed. Unapologetic*

Sisters of the Solstice Moon
(Book 1 of the When She Wakes series)

Gina Martin

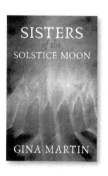

On the Winter Solstice, thirteen women across the world see the same terrifying vision. Their world is about to experience ravaging destruction. All that is now sacred will be destroyed. Each answers the call, to journey to Egypt, and save the wisdom of the Goddess.

She who is Kali Ma from the jungles of Arya, Tiamet from the Roof of the World, Badh of the Cailleach from the land of Eiru, Awa from the Land of Yemaya, Uxua of Ix Chel from the Yucatan, Parasfahe from the Land of Inanna...all racing against time and history to bring us their story.

An imagining... or is it a remembering... of the end of matriarchy and the emergence of global patriarchy, this book brings alive long dead cultures from around the world and brings us closer to the lost wisdoms that we know in our bones.

Printed in Great Britain
by Amazon

48714270R00130